Born Broken

Born Broken

DE-PATHOLOGIZING THE HUMAN CONDITION

DR. MATT RUSHFORD

ISBN-13: 9781512356182
ISBN-10: 1512356182

Acknowledgments

This book would have been impossible without the support and encouragement of my wife, Julieta. I would also like to thank all my friends, family, and practice members who never let me forget I promised them this book. Many of the concepts, philosophies, and lessons I have documented here are gleaned from generations of teachers who have come before me, from B.J. Palmer to Reggie Gold, Donny Epstein, Arno Burnier, Marsden Wagner, Suzanne Arms, Ina May Gaskin, and many, many others to whom I am eternally grateful.

For my parents, Don and Kathie Rushford

Contents

"We are all on edge. Human beings feel safe and secure when they can stand confidently in the center of things, either in the center of an age or in the center of a class of people with a common world-view, but when they come to an edge, they feel nervous and unsettled. There at the edge we see familiar things end and something else begin, something which makes us try to recall another state of being..."

-WILLIAM IRWIN THOMPSON, *THE TIME FALLING BODIES TAKE TO LIGHT*

Introduction

The idea for writing this book came from my experiences as a family chiropractor, a lecturer, and an instructor of anatomy and physiology. In each role, I found myself spending a surprising amount of time helping patients or students recognize and understand the difference between normal body parts and functions and abnormal expressions of biology.

For example, it consistently comes as a shock for students to learn that their tonsils, of which we actually have five, as well as their appendix, are made up of a type of tissue called "lymphoid tissue" that has a critical immunological role in the body. Both the appendix and tonsils house B and T lymphocytes, which help fight infections and even cancer, and the appendix is now known to be a source for recolonization of crucial gut bacteria (Chapter 19). You can hardly blame the students: The dissection video I show in class features a narration that includes the statement: "...the appendix is a vestigial but potentially troublesome organ..."

This reframing of normal to abnormal has been adopted as common knowledge. On a larger scale, we are left with the prevalent notion that the human body is intrinsically incompetent—that we are "born broken." In fact, quite the opposite is true. Every day, our bodies show us evidence of their intelligence and competence, even as we actively work against our bodies' efforts. The body does not always speak in languages that are comfortable or convenient, but for the overwhelming majority of us, we are not born broken.

In my chiropractic practice, my patients are often surprised to learn that there is intelligence in their low back pain or swollen joints. Understanding this intelligence is like a key that unlocks untapped potentialities in the healing process. And of course, a big part of the patient education process for our pregnant patients, including and especially the dads, is helping them to understand that a pregnant woman is not sick, even though virtually every element of most women's prenatal care encourages her to think she is.

As a lecturer, I've been invited to present this information at medical schools, hospitals, universities, colleges, seminars, symposiums, and other venues. And while I truly love the energy and personal experience of a live lecture or one-on-one discussion, I am constantly asked if I have this information in book form so that it can be shared and processed more easily. So, here it is.

As I researched for my classes and lectures, and even for this book, I encountered more and more examples of normal body processes that had somehow been re-framed in popular opinion as pathological, or sick, a process I came to call by the rather ungainly title, "Pathologization." Yes, it's awkward, but, hey, so is "photosynthesis." In some cases, the process of "De-Pathologizing" these concepts in the classroom was a long and arduous one. The "legs" of the ideological table that formed the distorted belief system had to be knocked off, logically, one by one before the person could reconsider their preconceptions. In other cases, it was just a simple question or analogy that flicked on the light switch.

The concept of Pathologization is, also, by no means one that I originated. You can find references to the Pathologization of childhood, women's bodies, sadness, anxiety, and countless other "normal" phenomena. The fact that Pathologization essentially monetizes these phenomena makes it a central talking point in circles ranging from psychiatry to pediatrics to women's health.

What causes Pathologization? As I researched for this book, I found cases in which Pathologization was clearly an intentional device, used to promote or elevate a profession or its agenda. After all, re-framing normal, healthy body functions or parts as abnormal is a powerful tool to engender dependence on those who possess the skill set to treat disease. Re-framing the normal into the abnormal also represents substantial new revenue sources for those entities. For the most part, however, I have come to believe that Pathologization is simply a by-product of the superimposition of the limited skill set of the physician within the vast and complex realm of human health. One sees what one wants to see; or, perhaps more accurately, one sees what one is trained to see.

Yet, Pathologization has real consequences. It promotes over-utilization of intervention and thus drives up health care costs and increases the risk of medical errors and damaging side-effects. Reframing pregnancy as a medical condition empowers clinicians to apply "preventive" measures like fetal monitoring and IV tubes, which have not been shown to improve outcomes and instead set into motion a cascade of interventions that, for one out of three American women, culminate in a major abdominal surgery.

Pathologization contributes to a general sense of impotence and a growing sense of fatalism about health and disease. Epidemiologists are spending less and less time (and our money) searching for the cause of disease and more and more time developing expensive and harmful treatments.

Pathologization enhances both dependence on allopathic medicine and a degree of abdication of responsibility for one's own health destiny. If no one is driving the car, what good are checking the oil and tire pressure going to do? Instead of soliciting our body's own innate potential for health, we are encouraged to simply watch and wait for the impending disaster and limit the damage when it inevitably occurs.

Conversely, De-Pathologizing the human body is a radical act of self-determinism. Dispelling mythologies about our bodies, which have falsely led us to believe we are weak, fragile, and perpetually in need of heroic intervention, is part of the larger process of empowerment and responsibility. This book is partly about the vestigial legends of the body and partly a celebration of the even greater truth. As the poet said, the Truth will set you free. Freedom is something that lives inside each of us.

As a chiropractor, I have the privilege of working in a community of practitioners and patients who are all living on the margins of the mainstream medical ecosystem, all searching for a deeper connection to the human experience of living and healing. My wife and I have had the great honor and blessing to help guide and enable this transformation, not only through the chiropractic adjustment, but through an ongoing dialogue about health which includes dispelling the mythology of Pathologization. When we dispel fallacies of our own faulty design, we are empowered to take on the task of being fully alive with greater responsibility and self-determinism. This process is not exclusive to chiropractic patients and yoginis; it is available to anyone who is willing to reconsider the fundamental nature of their body and the people who help it. Ultimately, this reawakening will reverse-percolate upwards to the larger systems that support these paradigms.

Re-writing the U.S. Health Care system is a task for brighter minds than mine, but I do hope to offer a course-correction—an observation about the limitations of our current paradigm and a series of examples of grass-roots actions and behaviors that can be part of a larger change in a more positive direction for all of us.

I've organized the book into three sections. The first is a discussion of health, medicine, and our medical delivery system, which we call "Health Care." Understanding the elemental nature of each of these subjects is critical in order to appreciate the paradigm shift that is happening as it relates specifically to the topics covered in the rest of the book.

Part Two is about Birth. Why have I dedicated so much of this book to the topics of pregnancy and childbirth? Because of all the aspects of the human condition that have been Pathologized, childbirth represents by far the most successful and most profoundly embedded reframing of normal into abnormal. Birth has become so deeply and unquestioningly Pathologized that even suggesting its normalcy is considered a radical act, and the history of that Pathologization is so old and muddled, the untangling process requires journeying back, quite literally, to the dawn of civilization.

In Part Three, I explore other examples of Pathologization, and bring the whole discussion into a context that allows you to take positive action with this information and make substantive changes in the way you see your body and engage with the Health Care system.

CHAPTER 1
Medicine, Health, and Disease

Introduction: Medicine that Works

William McCallister looks pretty much like any other 8-year-old kid in my practice. A little on the short side, perhaps, but otherwise he is a strapping, healthy, handsome kid who roughhouses with his older brother constantly, plays soccer, and loves Star Wars. By looking at him, you'd never know his secret—a past filled with peril, pain, and, literally, heartbreak. Unless, he took off his shirt.

Then you'd see the scar. Scars, actually. One big one running straight down his chest; others running laterally across his upper torso. These scars take up a majority of the skin on his chest. And they tell a different story.

You see, Billy was born with a congenital heart malformation called Hypoplastic Left Heart Syndrome, or HLHS. This is a condition in which the left side of the heart—the side that pumps blood to just about the entire body—is underdeveloped. At first, the baby may seem normal because the blood can get to the body through an opening called the ductus arteriosus. But soon this duct closes, and the child will become pale and have difficulty breathing. Until recently, there was no treatment for HLHS. Parents of these children were doomed to watch their child slowly just…fade away.

In 1979, a series of operations were developed to correct HLHS.[1] The concept is staggeringly bold: blood returning from the body, rather than entering the right side of the heart to be pumped to the lungs, would be sent directly to the lungs by connecting the venae cavae to the pulmonary arteries. Then blood returning from the lungs would be shunted to the right side of the heart, which would then be hooked up to the aorta, the main artery leaving the heart. So, essentially, the right side of the heart, which normally delivers blood to the lungs and is thus far smaller and weaker than the left, is now pumping blood to the entire body, and blood must reach the lungs by residual pressure in the system, rather than being sent to the heart first for a fresh push outwards. That the system can accommodate such a dramatic shift in demand while also adapting to the radical surgeries themselves, all within the age of three, is a testament to the staggering capacity of the human body. That medical science has developed the means to accomplish this procedure with any kind of safety is an equally impressive statement.

Today, the surgical correction of HLHS is associated with a 70%, 5 year survival rate.[2] That's up from zero. Billy McCallister is one of those lucky 70%, and his parents are among those very lucky people who can hug and kiss and hold their child every day thanks to the brilliant minds who developed this daring procedure.

I begin my discussion of the deep problems with medical science with this story for a good reason. It is to highlight the essence of what is *right* with today's Western medical model. It is an example of medical science, a powerful and specific tool, being used in the appropriate way, for the appropriate people, with clear and defendable results. Emergency medicine is another example of western medicine at its finest. Our first-response teams, emergency room staff, and critical care facilities represent, for the most part, the apex of science applied with appropriate respect to the relationship between the tool and the trade.

This book is not an excoriation of medicine, but rather a celebration of medical science and a reminder of the importance of using its gifts appropriately, wisely, and with restraint. For just like any other valuable, expensive tool, it can be used inappropriately, and with poor results.

In order to understand the origins of Pathologization and the impact it has on our society, we need to understand the nature of the milieu in which it operates: the U.S. Health Care System.

"Health Care" in the U.S. is not just big business; it's the biggest business.

Health care is the largest industry in the U.S. According to *Forbes* magazine,[3] U.S. health care spending reached $2.7 trillion in 2012, representing 17.3% of the nation's Gross National Product. The healthcare sector's rising share of the economy, magnified by a contraction in other sectors, reached 17.3 percent of the gross domestic product and is expected to reach 19.3 percent of GDP by the end of the decade.[4]

It is comprised of:

- hospitals
- medical doctors
- nurses
- other medical support staff
- physical therapists
- pharmacists
- lab technicians

Forty percent of all health care workers are employed by hospitals. The overwhelming majority of our interaction with our "Health Care System" involves engaging with medical doctors, nurses, physician assistants, and other medical professionals. So it's important to recognize that when we use the term "health care," we are actually talking about *medical care.*

U.S. HEALTH CARE = MEDICAL CARE

Why is this distinction important? Aren't these two things, health care and medical care, synonymous? You may be surprised at the answer.

These distinctions are important because the nature and parameters of medical care establish the paradigm within which we perceive ourselves, our bodies, and our health. How medicine sees us is, to a large degree, how we see ourselves. What may come as a surprise to many of you is how remarkably narrow the lens that medicine uses to view and consider the human body is.

So let's examine both medical care and human health. Then we'll look at them side by side and see if what we have been taught to believe about both holds true.

Medicine

Medicine is a branch of applied sciences that falls under the larger domain of natural science. It is a limited-scope specialty with limited clinical tools. The focus is limited to the treatment and prevention of symptoms and disease, and its tools are largely limited to drugs, radiation, and surgery (though emerging tools include genetic manipulation and nanotechnology).

From the Oxford Dictionary[5]:
Definition of **medicine**
noun
[*mass noun*]

1.   the science or practice of the diagnosis, treatment, and prevention of disease
2.   a drug or other preparation for the treatment or prevention of disease:

Medicine, by definition, focuses on disease.

Not only is medicine's clinical focus oriented around disease, but its educational focus is also similarly aligned. The truth is that modern medical doctors receive little training in the elements of human health and wellness. The optimal, fully empowered state of the human being and how to elicit that state are topics which are not really a part of medical training.

Different medical schools offer different combinations of classes in each phase of their education. However, most begin with classes in basic sciences, anatomy, physiology, biochemistry, etc. As the student progresses, they progress quickly to pathology, or the study of disease. Pathology, diagnosis, and the treatment of disease comprise an overwhelming majority of a typical medical school's training for doctors. Figure 13 shows the curriculum for the prestigious Emory School of Medicine.[6] The first four months of a doctor's long and arduous road to practice features, amidst intensive studies of basic and clinical sciences like biochemistry and anatomy, topics such as "nutrition" and "exercise." The title of this section is "Healthy Human." After four months of this, the curriculum then shifts to the section entitled, "Human Disease." This section lasts for a full year, and is followed by reviews, exams, and applications.

The visual effect of this educational strategy is a remarkably graphic illustration of the relative focus, in medicine, on health versus the focus on disease.

Emory School of Medicine Curriculum

At UT Southwestern Medical School, future doctors begin their studies with courses in basic sciences[7]: Anatomy, Biochemistry, Cell Biology, Embryology, Genetics, Human Behavior, Immunology, Neuroscience.

In their second year, the curriculum continues with anatomy and physiology with a shift towards pathology.

In the third year, students begin the first of two years of intense clinical training and experiences involving direct patient care. Rotations include:

- Family Medicine
- Internal Medicine
- Neurology
- Obstetrics and Gynecology
- Pediatrics
- Psychiatry
- Surgery

The fourth year consists of four-week clinical rotations. Four, four-week electives are chosen to fulfill the remaining course requirements.

- Acute Care Clerkship (*4 weeks*)
- Ambulatory Care Clerkship (*4 weeks*)
- Sub-internship (*4 weeks*)
- Four Electives (*4 weeks each*)

You may ask, if good health is primarily influenced by proper nutrition, exercise, and other lifestyle elements, where is the training and education in these subjects? The answer is, for medical students, it normally does not exist, and that is because those subjects are technically outside the scope of the practice of medicine.

The limited nature of the scope of medical education and treatment is critical to appreciate, because, while we use the term "health care" to describe what M.D.s provide, in reality, doctors only address one small element of human health, namely, whether we have diseases or not. Yet avoiding disease is only one small part of being healthy.

When you walk into a doctor's office, the basic clinical questions they have are simple:

1. What is your chief complaint (your symptoms)?
2. What is your condition, if any (your diagnosis)?
3. What is our recommended treatment, or referral?
4. What is your prognosis?

Try walking into a doctor's office and saying, "I don't have any symptoms or illnesses, and don't want to be checked for any. I just want my health cared for." What is there for that doctor to do? What training has he or she received to prepare them to treat you in this respect? If you're lucky, they may perhaps give you some suggestions in terms of diet, or exercise or weight loss that are oriented around avoiding diabetes, heart disease, or other illnesses. However, as there are few insurance codes or reimbursement for this type of interaction, it is simply not supported by the "health care system" infrastructure.

At its essence, medical care is ultimately a limited field specialty focusing on those rare periods of crisis in which we are faced with trauma, illness, or other symptom-generating problems.

Yet we don't use medicine in a limited way.

"Remember, we are creatures of popular culture, we revere doctors as if they were the heroes and heroines we grew up watching on T.V. It's the doctors who are so honorably portrayed on everything from Dr. Kildare to Dr. Quinn, Medicine Woman."

-The Girlfriend's Guide to Pregnancy[8]

Medical doctors today enjoy a high level of prestige and social status. We trust our doctor. At any given time, doctors are featured in several different dramas on television and in the movies as intelligent authorities in matters of health and life in general. We associate doctors with affluence, wisdom, intelligence, and an almost superhuman capacity for objectivity and decisiveness. We have phrases in our lexicon like, "Trust me, I'm a doctor." We are told to "consult with our physician" before engaging in an exercise program, changing our diet, or getting pregnant, even though most M.D.s graduate from medical school with little to no training or education in exercise science, nutrition, or even normal pregnancy and birth.

In my hometown of Burlington, Vermont, a local pediatrician has regular advice forums in newspaper, radio, and even television stations. He offers advice on everything from helmet safety to sex education, barking dogs and even father's day gifts.

We assume he is an expert on these topics, regardless of the fact that there is nothing inherent in the education of a physician that would make him an "expert" in any of these fields. And while this particular gentleman is a sweet guy and his advice column contains some good information, it is, at the same time, naturally biased towards the medical/pathological perspective, which, while not illegitimate, is nevertheless very narrow.

The Advent of The Medical Monopoly

"Anything can deliver us from our loss of memory of the soul: science, history, art, or the sunlight on the grass tatami mats in the Zendo. And anything can enslave us: science, history, art, or the militarism of the Zen academy. But if we are lost in time and suffering from a racial amnesia, then we need something to startle us into recollection. If history is the sentence of our imprisonment, then history, recoded, can become the password of our release..."

- William Irwin Thompson, *The Time Falling Bodies Take to Light*

Many readers will be surprised to learn that allopathic medicine's current role as the sole arbiter of the vast, complex realm of human wellness is actually relatively new. In fact, not too long ago, the main role of a doctor was as a surgeon, and the notion that a medical doctor would be relied upon for advice or treatment in broader fields of health would have been absurd.

Understanding the history of that cultural change can help us to reassess our relationship to both medicine and our own bodies.

Most people would be surprised to discover that prior to the 20th century:

- Medical doctors occupied a low status in society.
- Medical care was dangerous, superstitious, ineffective, unscientific, untested, unproven, and often tortuous and barbaric.
- Most of medicine was based on concepts derived from writers of the 5th century BC that were not questioned for 2,000 years and have only relatively recently been debunked.
- Allopathic medicine achieved a monopoly over the health care industry through a calculated cultural appropriation whose success was based on successful political and social strategies, not superior scientific or clinical skills.

Historian Paul Starr won the Pulitzer Prize in 1984 for his seminal work on this subject, "The Social Transformation of American Medicine." Starr's work looked at how the medical profession in America rose from a "relatively weak, traditional profession of minor economic significance" to a position whose cultural and clinical authority extends into the realms of moral, economic, and political influence.

"Some may think the sources of professional sovereignty too obvious to be worth pursuing," Starr wrote. "For haven't healers always been esteemed and powerful? And doesn't the growth of science make inevitable the high value and position attached to medicine? And isn't there something about American culture, particularly our preoccupation with health and well-being, that makes us especially inclined to give doctors a high status? The answer to each of these questions is no."

For the majority of its existence, medicine has based its theory and practice on the writings of Hippocrates, who lived in Greece around 500 BC. His theories of "the Humors" of the body were adopted without question or scientific examination and remained the standard of medical theory until the 16th century, when the church began to release restrictions on cadaveric experimentation.

The tools of medicine remained largely superstitious and ineffective into the 1800s.

Edward Bergmark, PhD, is CEO of American Telecare and board member of the Chicago School of Professional Psychology. He recently described 18th century medicine:

"What we're going to do is go back a few years, back to when the average life span was 35 years, which gave people the opportunity to go through their teenage years and midlife at the same time. Back then, the standard treatment was bloodletting. During the yellow fever epidemic, Benjamin Rush, physician signator to the Declaration of Independence, bled 100 to 125 people per day. Also common at the time was purging, a treatment that had the benefit of visible results. Hanging was popular for some diseases, a case of iatrogenic disease taken to the extreme.

Other treatments, such as sweat boxes and mercury ointments, could be tortures as well to the patient. Prior to anesthesia, medicine was often a horror show. Patients died of shock during surgery. A doctor's greatest assets were strength and speed. According to the Guinness Book of World Records, one physician was clocked at doing a leg amputation below the hip at 33 seconds—even if he did once accidentally remove the fingers of three assistants during one surgery.

Doctors were helpless in the face of infection or fever. "Childbirth fever" was fatal for centuries, with a higher rate of death for deliveries in a hospital than at home. There is little wonder at this statistic, as a report from a particular French hospital recounts six patients in one bed, body pressed against body, suffering from various conditions, such as post-pregnancy, infantile disease, typhus, and severe skin rash. Prior to the 1800s, there were no facilities for washing hands before a procedure. Doctors would routinely go straight to an obstetrics patient from the necropsy room.

If you didn't take care of yourself and keep yourself out of the hospital back then, the price was indeed high."

Consider the contrast in the development of knowledge between medicine and the other sciences throughout history. At a time when the movements of the stars and planets could be tracked and predicted with astonishing accuracy, the laws of accelerated motion and parabolic trajectory had been described, and mathematical theorems and principles which are still valid and in use today were known (calculus was invented before the year 1700), the primary medical practices—all of which have since been soundly debunked—centered on bleeding, hanging, and purging and remained deeply entrenched in medicine into the 1800s.

Physicians, tragically, killed America's founding father himself. On December 12th, 1799, George Washington contracted a sore throat after remaining in cold, wet clothes for two days. His doctors purged his bowels with strong laxatives and removed an astonishing nine pints of blood from his body.[9] America's first hero died shortly afterwards.

The status of the American medical doctor, as recently as the early 20th century, was astonishingly poor.

"From the Jacksonian period through the end of the nineteenth century, a medical career did not carry the prestige and guaranteed security it does today. In 1832, J. Marion Sims, who would later become one of America's foremost surgeons, returned home to his family in South Carolina after graduating from college. His mother, who had recently died, had wanted him to become a clergyman; his father hoped he would become a lawyer. Sims wanted to be neither, and felt that if he had to take up a profession, medicine would make the fewest demands on his frail talents. 'If I had known this,' his father exclaimed in an outburst that might amuse parents today, 'I certainly should not have sent you to college… it is a profession for which I have the utmost contempt. There is no science in it. There is no honor to be achieved in it; no reputation to be made.' "[10]

As late as 1870, a medical journal remarked that when a young man of merit and ability chose to become a doctor "the feeling among the majority of his cultivated friends is that he has thrown himself away."

It is interesting to note that the specific inadequacies of a 19th century medical career are the exact aspects for which it is known today. This is at least partially because the techniques and results with which physicians were associated—bleeding, heavy doses of mercury, caustic, torturous methods which are now believed to range "from ineffective to lethal"—were indeed anything but scientific, but rather a compilation and codification of ancient, esoteric, and often mystical teachings which had never truly been subjected to rational examination or review, and would not be until the early 20th century.

Medical doctors at this time were not the only people in the "healing" business. Eastern Europe also was populated by herbalism, hydrotherapy, pharmacology, and, of course, the midwives who birthed virtually all of the children, and:

"...developed an extensive understanding of bones and muscles, herbs and drugs, while physicians were still deriving their prognoses from astrology and alchemists were trying to turn lead into gold."[11]

According to Starr, the emergence of the allopathic physician as the solitary authority in the realm of human health came about as a result of an organized social and political scheme that ultimately elevated the medical doctor in the absence of any significant scientific or clinical expertise.

He wrote:

"...In terms of medical skills and theory, the so-called "regulars" had nothing to recommend them over lay practitioners. Their "formal training" meant little even by European standards of the time. Medical programs varied in length from a few months to two years; many medical schools had no clinical facilities; high school diplomas were not required for admission to medical schools. Not that serious academic training would have helped much anyway—there was no body of medical science to be trained in. Instead, the "regulars" were taught to treat most ills by "heroic" measures: massive bleeding, huge doses of laxatives, calomel (a laxative containing mercury) and, later, opium.... The lay practitioners were undoubtedly safer and more effective than the "regulars." They preferred mild herbal medications, dietary changes, and hand-holding to heroic interventions... left alone, they might have displaced the medical doctors with even middle class consumers in time. But they didn't know the right people. The "regulars," with their close ties to the upper class, had legislative clout. By 1830, 13 states had passed medical licensing laws outlawing "irregular" practice and establishing "regulars" as the only legal healers."[12]

In 1846, the American Medical Association was formed. The two main components of its code were: 1) the elevation and standardization of requirements for medical degrees; and, 2) the denial of "fraternal courtesy" with "irregular" practitioners. In other words, the goal was to elevate the status of the physician and exclude alternative practitioners from the medical marketplace.

"... monopoly was doubtless the intent of the AMA's program..."[13]

Early attempts at gaining a monopoly were unsuccessful, according to Starr, because the American public balked at the establishment of a kind of professional ruling class, which held and withheld esoteric information from the public domain. The ultimate answer for the "regulars" was to actually open membership to their competitors, while simultaneously establishing codes of clinical conduct that made it impossible for them to thrive.

Another important act of facilitation for the medical doctors was the establishment of unusual rules of liability in the late nineteenth century. The courts set the standard of care as that of the local community where a physician practiced.

"This limited possible expert testimony against physicians to their immediate colleagues. By adopting the 'locality rule,' the courts prepared the way for granting considerable power to the local medical society, for it became almost impossible for patients to get testimony against a physician who was a member..."[14]

Successful suits against AMA physicians were virtually eliminated. This tacit immunity from legal recourse became an irresistible incentive for even more physicians to join the allegiance.

Still, effective therapeutic agents in medicine were few. Furthermore, medical knowledge was in many cases incomplete or patently incorrect. For example, the infant formulas promoted so vigorously by physicians in the late 19th century were gravely unhealthy, and resulted in much higher mortality rates for artificially-fed infants versus breastfed ones. Most doctors knew little about nutrition[15] and their recommendations were "unreliable." But medical authority, according to Starr, "was not necessarily weaker for being objectively incorrect."

"The growth of medical authority was related more to the success of science in revolutionizing other aspects of medicine and the growing recognition of the inadequacy of the unaided and uneducated senses in understanding the world."[16]

So in a sense the medical profession had not necessarily proven itself worthy of being granted its authority, except on the grounds that, as a member of a larger branch of scientific thought, it "rode the coattails" of the scientific revolution, which was by contrast demonstrating positive results in human health and welfare. Public health and hygiene measures, such as cleaner water, safer food, and waste disposal had massive impacts on health and disease.

Slate writer Laura Helmuth recently wrote a piece on longevity in the U.S. called "Why Are You Not Dead Yet?"[17]

"How did we go from the miseries of the past to our current expectation of long and healthy lives? "Most people credit medical advances," says David Jones, a medical historian at Harvard—"but most historians would not." One problem is the timing. Most of the effective medical treatments we recognize as saving our lives today have been available only since World War II: antibiotics, chemotherapy, drugs to treat high blood pressure. But the steepest increase in life expectancy occurred from the late 1800s to the mid-1900s.... **Clean water alone has been shown to be responsible for nearly half the total mortality reduction in major cities, three quarters of the infant mortality reduction, and nearly two thirds of the child mortality reduction in the U.S."**[18]

Historian Thomas McKeown's rather exhaustive analysis of the question of the role of medical advances in the reduction of mortality in eastern Europe in the last several hundred years led him to the same conclusion:

"(Medical) treatment contributed little to the reduction of deaths from infectious diseases before 1935, and over the period since the cause of death was first registered they were much less important than other influences..."[19]

McKinley and Mckinley's 1977 study of the same question in the U.S. resulted in the same conclusion.

"In general, medical measures (both chemotherapeutic and prophylactic) appear to have contributed little to the overall decline in mortality in the United States since about 1900—having in many instances been introduced several decades after a marked decline had already set in and mostly having no detectable influence...it is estimated that at most 3.5 percent of the total decline in mortality since 1900 could be ascribed to medical measures..."[20]

Meanwhile, the "detached technologies" of the stethoscope, ophthalmoscope, and laryngoscope enhanced the "persuasive rhetoric" of medical authority. Advancements in scientific understanding of anatomy, physiology, and other applications of medicine, though not translating to significantly improved patient outcomes relative to public health measures, did serve to improve the perceived relevance of the medical doctor.

"Cultural authority need not be based on competence. Ambiguity may suffice."[21]

The "retreat of private judgment" in which the scientific revolution in general, and the medical industry specifically participated, involved a larger social and political transformation. This involved what Starr calls "institutionalized dependence" and "lay deference": the abdication of personal judgment on the part of the public towards doctors. We agreed to "trust our doctor." By capitalizing on these changes, medicine was able to successfully achieve a virtual monopoly on health care in America and convince the public to cede their personal judgment in favor of that of medicine.

While the retreat of private judgment may be a necessary component of a larger social construct such as organized medicine, it still has conspicuous, inescapable risks. A lack of scrutiny and healthy skepticism can enable the perpetuation of dysfunctional protocols, politically motivated decisions, and what Marsden Wagner calls, "anti-precautionary medicine."

The result of what Starr calls "the social transformation of American medicine" was also the establishment of Western allopathic medicine as the sole presiding body for the entirety of the American health care system. The primary problem with this monopoly is that medicine, though greatly expanded both socially and culturally, remained, and remains today, a specialized field of clinical expertise. That area of specialization is the diagnosis and treatment of disease. But health as a whole is an objective, which involves far more than simply avoiding and eliminating disease. Medical training is simply inadequate to address it all.

More importantly, medicine may fail to take into consideration the very considerable capacities of the human body to restore and maintain health naturally. For solutions, doctors will naturally look at the problem through the lens of the tools available to them: drugs, radiation, and surgery. But these, like any tools, are limited, and not always the appropriate tool for the task at hand.

Medicine today, and more importantly, the medical paradigm, is being applied to a realm of human situations that is so far beyond its skill set that the only possible consequence is poor outcomes.

The value in appreciating the manner in which medicine advanced socially in America is in how it gives us an opportunity to re-examine our tacit agreement with doctors for "institutionalized dependence" and a "surrender of private judgment." These contracts were written over a century and a half ago, before Google, before PubMed, and before advancements in technology and our understanding of hygiene, health, and wellness empowered ordinary citizens to not only question their doctors with an unprecedented amount of information at their fingertips, but to assume a massive amount of power to create and maintain their own health, naturally, through diet, exercise, and other healthy lifestyle practices.

Understanding that the apotheosis of modern American medicine was not necessarily a reflection of its competence as a universal arbiter of the broad, complex realm of well-being allows us to reconsider the degree to which (or conditions under which) we will continue to defer to their social authority. Contextualizing medicine, appreciating the limitations of its field of expertise, allows us to set more responsible parameters for that deference. I would, for example, defer without question to the emergency room surgeon with lives hanging in the balance; with some questioning, but substantial deference, to the critical-care doctor managing a case of end-organ failure; and with respect but healthy skepticism to the general practitioner who insists that the best way for me to achieve health is to take blood-thinning drugs for the rest of my life.

MEDICAL CARE = DISEASE CARE

Contextualizing medicine means, for the first time, assigning boundaries around our relationship with doctors that are congruent with the clinical limitations of medicine itself. The result is to maximize the substantial gifts and benefits of allopathy while confronting the poor outcomes that can result from the incongruence between western medicine and health care. Most importantly, this opens the door for a new relationship with our own bodies in which the process of De-Pathologization engenders a renewed sense of trust in our innate healing capacity.

The problem with using medicine for health care is that medicine is actually better described as a disease/crisis management system, though at its best, it is a superlative one.

The Mind of a Surgeon & The Handy Hammer

My father-in-law, a world-famous kidney transplant surgeon and a personal hero and mentor, once described his analytical approach to handling a patient in crisis. He said, "Mateo, the first thing I do, is I think, what is the worst thing that could happen at this moment to this patient?" On a scrap of napkin he then draws the beginning of a marvelously complex flow chart. "And the next thing I do is I create an action plan to respond to this potential event, a series of responses, including actions I could take to prevent the event from taking place at all. Next, I think, what if all of these actions fail? And I come up with fallback responses to that contingency. Then, I think, okay, what is the NEXT worst thing that could happen to this patient? And I continue on this course until I have established a kind of flow chart based on the most likely emergency and the response most likely to prevent or correct it."

I found this a fascinating view into the mind of a gifted doctor. It is what I call "Anti-Trust" mentality: We don't just trust or hope that these bad things will not happen because they are actually imminent possibilities. In emergency medicine, it is dangerous to assume that bad things won't happen. I think it's safe to say that this mindset is descriptive of most surgeons, if not most medical doctors. Anti-Trust is, in fact, the elemental mindset of medicine itself. The practice of medicine was borne out of and remains a field which is perpetually on alert for threats to the safety of the human body.

More importantly, I would suggest that it is exactly the kind of thinking that any of us would want our doctor using if we were in a life-threatening situation: massive trauma from a car accident or end stage organ failure, cardiovascular emergency, etc. At these moments, the body is under highly unusual conditions: It has been compromised and is in emergency mode. The limitations of its physical matter have been exceeded. In these moments, to simply "trust" that the body will take care of itself is reckless and potentially catastrophic. Employing the kind of "Anti-Trust" mentality described above is the appropriate choice in emergency situations. It is just what I want my doctor to do if my body is in crisis and struggling to keep me alive.

The interesting question, and one we will spend more time exploring in this book is: What happens when we apply this Anti-Trust strategy to ALL moments of human health, not just special emergency situations? Is it appropriate to NEVER trust the human body to heal itself or conduct everyday functions?

Why would medical doctors tend to not trust the body? Medical doctors see the world through the lens of disease. So it is natural that a medical doctor will look at almost any aspect of human physiology through the lens of disease. It's called the Handy Hammer phenomenon. When all you've got is a hammer, everything looks like a nail. But it's ridiculous to view *every* aspect of the body as pathological. Does medicine do this? We are going to investigate that question in depth in this book and look to see that the Handy Hammer effect has actually developed in medicine to the point that not only are humans considered intrinsically pathological or "Born Broken," but even nature itself has to some degree become re-framed as pathological.

Integrative and functional medicine pioneer, Dr. Frank Lipman, M.D., wrote in the Huffington Post:

"The problem is that although most of us are not permanently in a health "crisis," this crisis care model is being used to treat our every health problem or symptom as if it is the only health care model we have. Most of us are not sick enough to be in hospital, and by far the majority of people who visit their doctor, do so for ongoing chronic problems like diabetes, heart disease, and obesity, or less-defined ailments like joint pains, back pains, fatigue, and headaches. Western medicine's solutions to these problems are drugs and surgery."[22]

So, when we look at the true nature of modern medicine, we do have to ask ourselves: Is the prevention and treatment of diseases all there is to optimal human health? I believe the answer to that question is a resounding NO. And that answer depends on a working definition of health.

What is Health?

The question we are asking is, does being healthy equate to the absence of symptoms and disease?

The World Health Organization doesn't think so.

It defines health as, "a state of complete physical, mental, and social well-being and not merely the absence of disease or infirmity."[23]

Dr. Guy Reikman, president of Life University and author of *The Power of One* describes it this way:

"If they could magically come up with a way to end all disease on earth, I'd be first in line. But even then, that wouldn't mean we would suddenly be healthy, any more than ending divorce would suddenly mean that everyone had happy marriages. I'm sure many of you know someone who is married, NOT divorced, but is not at all happy. That's because happiness in marriage is much, much more than simply NOT being divorced. And health is correspondingly much, much more than simply NOT having illness or symptoms."[24]

Curing, treating, or even preventing disease does not equate to health simply because being healthy means more than simply not being ill.

While it may be true that being healthy is difficult when one has a sickness or disease, it is also true that health is about far more than whether you are sick or not.

True health is something that involves every aspect of our human condition in the physical, mental, emotional, and spiritual realm. For example, our mental health affects our physical health. If you are depressed, your body expresses physical manifestations of that depression. In fact, chronic mental depression carries with it physical risks of illness and disease, like heart disease.[25]

We can include social health on our list of factors impacting physical health and wellness. Studies have shown that a person's feeling of connection and support with and from others influences their physical health. A famous study was accidentally conducted at the University of Houston, which was attempting to measure the effects of a high cholesterol diet on the development of atherosclerosis (blocked arteries). Genetically similar rabbits were all given feed high in cholesterol and all the rabbits developed atherosclerosis except one group. The mystery deepened when investigators discovered that all the healthy rabbits were kept in the same row of cages about four feet off the floor. This made no sense to the scientists until they discovered that the lab technician, who was short, would take these rabbits out of their cages at night when she came in to feed them. She would pet them and kiss them and return them to their cages. Rates of atherosclerosis were 60 percent lower in the nurtured group, even though they were given the same diet, and in fact *even had the same blood cholesterol levels, heart rate, and blood pressure.*[26]

Studies have repeatedly shown that social isolation increases the risk of heart disease and lowers immune function, independently of age, smoking, alcohol intake, and degree of emotional stress.[27] Physical exercise, spiritual health, and mental attitude all have been similarly shown to be important factors in overall health.

On a deeper level, these factors—social, emotional, spiritual, mental, physical, physiological, etc.—contribute to health in a dynamic way independent of the progression of illness and disease, or even symptoms. Let's call this deeper consideration "well-being."

The CDC says[28]:

Researchers from different disciplines have examined different aspects of well-being that include the following:

- *Physical well-being.*

- *Economic well-being.*
- *Social well-being.*
- *Development and activity.*
- *Emotional well-being.*
- *Psychological well-being.*
- *Life satisfaction.*
- *Domain specific satisfaction.*
- *Engaging activities and work.*

The University of Minnesota's Center for Spirituality and Healing has the concept of well-being at its core (they use the term "Wellbeing").

Here's how they define it:

"Wellbeing is a state of balance or alignment in body, mind, and spirit. In this state, we feel content; connected to purpose, people and community; peaceful and energized; resilient and safe. In short, we are flourishing."[29]

Their model, developed by Mary Jo Kreitzer, PhD, RN, FAAN, identifies six core elements to Wellbeing:

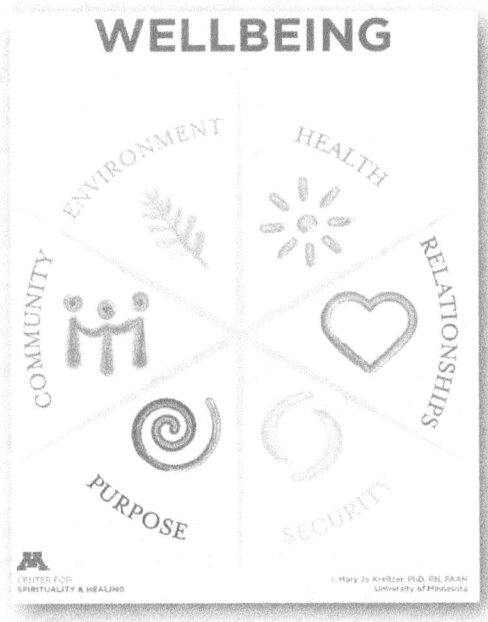

Health, Relationships, Environment, Community, Purpose, and Security.

This multidimensional view of human health is not the product of an intellectual exercise, it is simply an affirmation of what should be obvious: The human condition is inescapably multidimensional. Human health is an expression of the state of the human condition; therefore, human health is multidimensional. And when we affirm this complexity, we are affirming all elements of it, including those that we may not know how to measure or enhance effectively yet.

The term "well-being" is just a way of describing "health" in a way that escapes the narrow medical interpretation that has accompanied the term and acknowledges its intrinsic, multifaceted nature. The bottom line is that we humans are multifaceted, multilayered creatures and our ultimate satisfaction in life is a complex equation involving factors that range from linear to esoteric. Well-being supersedes the parameters of sickness and disease. One may be free from illness and have a very low level of well-being; one may have a serious illness and actually have a high level of well-being. In fact, in some cases, the illness itself is the very catalyst for the transformation of well-being. This is called "post-traumatic growth."

Psychology Today's Steve Taylor writes:

"Of all diseases, the one that is most likely to bring post-traumatic growth is cancer. It's because of this that survivors of cancer sometimes talk about the illness in almost spiritual terms, as a "great teacher" or even a gift. [One patient] who survived testicular cancer at the age of 25 has said that since having cancer, he has become "more complete, compassionate, and more intelligent, and therefore more alive."[30]

Health Insurance

Unfortunately, today, when we talk about "health care," we are really talking about medical care, which is care for sickness and disease. And when we use the term "health care system," we are really just talking about *insurance for medical care.*

Health insurance, as a kind of wholesale outlet for medical treatment, is organized emphatically around the medical paradigm, that is, around the administration of palliative and curative care. For example, even as a chiropractor, if I want to work with insurance, I must fill out a form that looks like this:

| 1500 |
| HEALTH INSURANCE CLAIM FORM |
| APPROVED BY NATIONAL UNIFORM CLAIM COMMITTEE 08/05 |

PICA ‖ ‖ ‖

CARRIER

| 1. MEDICARE (Medicare #) | MEDICAID (Medicaid #) | TRICARE CHAMPUS (Sponsor's SSN) | CHAMPVA (Member ID#) | GROUP HEALTH PLAN (SSN or ID) | FECA BLK LUNG (SSN) | OTHER (ID) | 1a. INSURED'S I.D. NUMBER (For Program in Item 1) |

| 2. PATIENT'S NAME (Last Name, First Name, Middle Initial) | 3. PATIENT'S BIRTH DATE MM DD YY   SEX M F | 4. INSURED'S NAME (Last Name, First Name, Middle Initial) |

| 5. PATIENT'S ADDRESS (No., Street) | 6. PATIENT RELATIONSHIP TO INSURED Self Spouse Child Other | 7. INSURED'S ADDRESS (No., Street) |

| CITY | STATE | 8. PATIENT STATUS Single Married Other | CITY | STATE |

| ZIP CODE | TELEPHONE (Include Area Code) (   ) | Employed Full-Time Student Part-Time Student | ZIP CODE | TELEPHONE (Include Area Code) (   ) |

PATIENT AND INSURED INFORMATION

| 9. OTHER INSURED'S NAME (Last Name, First Name, Middle Initial) | 10. IS PATIENT'S CONDITION RELATED TO: | 11. INSURED'S POLICY GROUP OR FECA NUMBER |

| a. OTHER INSURED'S POLICY OR GROUP NUMBER | a. EMPLOYMENT? (Current or Previous) YES NO | a. INSURED'S DATE OF BIRTH MM DD YY   SEX M F |

| b. OTHER INSURED'S DATE OF BIRTH MM DD YY   SEX M F | b. AUTO ACCIDENT? YES NO   PLACE (State) | b. EMPLOYER'S NAME OR SCHOOL NAME |

| c. EMPLOYER'S NAME OR SCHOOL NAME | c. OTHER ACCIDENT? YES NO | c. INSURANCE PLAN NAME OR PROGRAM NAME |

| d. INSURANCE PLAN NAME OR PROGRAM NAME | 10d. RESERVED FOR LOCAL USE | d. IS THERE ANOTHER HEALTH BENEFIT PLAN? YES NO   If yes, return to and complete item 9 a-d. |

READ BACK OF FORM BEFORE COMPLETING & SIGNING THIS FORM.

| 12. PATIENT'S OR AUTHORIZED PERSON'S SIGNATURE I authorize the release of any medical or other information necessary to process this claim. I also request payment of government benefits either to myself or to the party who accepts assignment below. SIGNED _____ DATE _____ | 13. INSURED'S OR AUTHORIZED PERSON'S SIGNATURE I authorize payment of medical benefits to the undersigned physician or supplier for services described below. SIGNED _____ |

| 14. DATE OF CURRENT: ILLNESS (First symptom) OR MM DD YY INJURY (Accident) OR PREGNANCY(LMP) | 15. IF PATIENT HAS HAD SAME OR SIMILAR ILLNESS. GIVE FIRST DATE MM DD YY | 16. DATES PATIENT UNABLE TO WORK IN CURRENT OCCUPATION MM DD YY   MM DD YY FROM   TO |

| 17. NAME OF REFERRING PROVIDER OR OTHER SOURCE | 17a. 17b. NPI | 18. HOSPITALIZATION DATES RELATED TO CURRENT SERVICES MM DD YY   MM DD YY FROM   TO |

| 19. RESERVED FOR LOCAL USE | 20. OUTSIDE LAB? YES NO $ CHARGES |

| 21. DIAGNOSIS OR NATURE OF ILLNESS OR INJURY (Relate Items 1, 2, 3 or 4 to Item 24E by Line) 1. ____ 3. ____ 2. ____ 4. ____ | 22. MEDICAID RESUBMISSION CODE   ORIGINAL REF. NO. |
| | 23. PRIOR AUTHORIZATION NUMBER |

24. A. DATE(S) OF SERVICE		B. PLACE OF SERVICE	C. EMG	D. PROCEDURES, SERVICES, OR SUPPLIES (Explain Unusual Circumstances) CPT/HCPCS MODIFIER	E. DIAGNOSIS POINTER	F. $ CHARGES	G. DAYS OR UNITS	H. EPSDT Family Plan	I. ID. QUAL	J. RENDERING PROVIDER ID. #
From MM DD YY	To MM DD YY									
1									NPI	
2									NPI	
3									NPI	
4									NPI	
5									NPI	
6									NPI	

PHYSICIAN OR SUPPLIER INFORMATION

| 25. FEDERAL TAX I.D. NUMBER SSN EIN | 26. PATIENT'S ACCOUNT NO. | 27. ACCEPT ASSIGNMENT? (For govt. claims, see back) YES NO | 28. TOTAL CHARGE $ | 29. AMOUNT PAID $ | 30. BALANCE DUE $ |

| 31. SIGNATURE OF PHYSICIAN OR SUPPLIER INCLUDING DEGREES OR CREDENTIALS (I certify that the statements on the reverse apply to this bill and are made a part thereof.) SIGNED _____ DATE _____ | 32. SERVICE FACILITY LOCATION INFORMATION a.   b. | 33. BILLING PROVIDER INFO & PH # (   ) a.   b. |

NUCC Instruction Manual available at: www.nucc.org   APPROVED OMB-0938-0999 FORM CMS-1500 (08-05)

Most of the form is bureaucratic red tape, but the salient point lies in the question of what is being treated. Question 10 reads:

IS PATIENT'S **CONDITION** RELATED TO:
EMPLOYMENT   AUTO ACCIDENT   OTHER ACCIDENT

It goes on to ask the onset of the current illness, injury or pregnancy and the diagnosis and nature of the current illness or injury. These are the only options available. There are no spaces for Wellbeing enhancement or optimization of Human Potential. This speaks to the specific and limited nature of the relationship that we are engaged in: illness, injury, symptoms, diagnosis, and treatment.

Using "health insurance" for "health care" is predicated on illness or injury. There is no space on this form for health maintenance, illness prevention, proactive measures, or quality of life, or human performance enhancement. The form asks for the diagnosis of the illness or injury and insists that each procedural code be matched with a specific medical diagnostic code related to that illness or injury.

Health insurance is wholly devoted to supporting the objectives of allopathic medicine: the diagnosis, treatment, and prevention of disease. Whether you're a chiropractor or medical doctor or any other kind of health care provider, you use forms like this every day if you work "in the system." (This is why I don't work "in the system.") Reimbursement for services, and thus the services themselves, are explicitly related to the treatment of conditions, injuries, and illnesses. If you continue treatment of the condition beyond a specific point, you must file forms which demonstrate "medical justification for continuation of care," which means you must show why the person's illness still requires treatment.

Together, the medical profession and medical care insurance combine to form a system oriented purely around detecting, categorizing, and treating symptoms, trauma, and diseases.

U.S. HEALTH CARE SYSTEM = INSURANCE CARE SYSTEM = DISEASE CARE SYSTEM

The fact that our health care system is really just a disease care system is not a new observation. It is a reality that has been noted by many critics in the past, including doctors themselves.

Edward Bergmark, biotechnology innovator who earlier gave us such a graphic depiction of 18th century medicine, also commented on 21st century medicine, saying, "We don't have health care in this country. We have sick care. We're completely out of balance."[31]

Integrative Medicine pioneer and author Dr. Andrew Weil has spoken out about this difference between health care and disease care.

"I have argued for years that we do not have a health care system in America. We have a disease-management system—one that depends on ruinously expensive drugs and surgeries that treat health conditions after they manifest rather than give our citizens simple diet, lifestyle, and therapeutic tools to keep them healthy," he wrote.[32]

Dr. Lipman adds:

"Although we talk about a 'health care' system and health care reform, what we're actually talking about is a 'disease care' system and disease care reform. Doctors of modern Western medicine are trained to treat disease with drugs and surgery. They are not trained to keep people healthy.

At medical school, we doctors are taught how to treat the symptoms of disease, rather than how to prevent disease in the first place. For example, throughout our training we receive very few lectures on nutrition, despite the fact that diet is fundamental to good health. Nor are we trained in other lifestyle modalities that help keep people well, such as exercise and relaxation therapies. We are taught nothing about the wisdoms of alternative medical systems that have been helping other cultures for centuries..."

DISEASE CARE ≠ HEALTH CARE

Understanding the difference between health care and disease care will help us to understand the dangers of confusing them.

How is "disease care" not an adequate expression of "health care?"

In order to understand the difference, all we have to do is look at what the terms "Health" and "Disease" actually mean in the real world of human biology. I've introduced the idea that "Health" is something more than simply not "being sick."

"Disease" as a concept may seem fairly straightforward:

Definition of **disease**
    noun

- a disorder of structure or function in a human, animal, or plant, especially one that produces specific symptoms or that affects a specific location and is not simply a direct result of physical injury:
  -Oxford Dictionary 2012[33]

So, disease or illness refers to an abnormality of structure or function in the body. But mostly it is predicated by the presence of detectable symptoms or signs. In other words, we don't consider ourselves ill until the illness has been detected.

I recall years ago when President George H. W. Bush was in office, a radio news report made the following statement:

"President Bush became ill yesterday when doctors detected an irregularity in his heart..."

The unspoken assumption in the phrasing of that report was that, until his irregularity was detected, he was perfectly fine. In reality, we know that this was not at all true for the president, nor is it true for many organic disturbances, as we will see a little later on.

For the purposes of this part of our journey, we can simply establish that when we are talking about "disease" or "illness," we are really talking about overt, measurable, identifiable symptoms and signs (like blood work lab values, vital sign abnormalities, orthopedic or neurological tests, etc.). This distinction is important because in fact so many illnesses and diseases spend the majority of their progression and do the majority of their damage without generating any measurable symptoms or signs.

For example, we can have no measurable illness or disease and be very, very sick.

- For 50% of people who suffer a heart attack, their first warning symptom is death; 300,000 to 400,000 Americans a year die in this way.[34]
- Many cancers, such as ovarian, pancreatic, lung, and breast, have been shown to develop free from symptoms for the vast majority of their ultimate progression, bringing the victim to within a hair's breadth of death before showing any conspicuous signs.[35]
- Physical fitness is not even a sign of health. Jim Fixx, the author of *The Complete Book of Running* and lifelong avid distance runner, died of heart failure *while running* at age 52.[36] (Fixx actually died in my home state of Vermont, in a town called Hardwick).
- Sean Eliot, star forward for the San Antonio Spurs in the 1990s, hit the play-off series-winning 3-point shot that sent his team to the championship,

which they won. Only weeks later, he announced that he needed a kidney transplant to live. The annals of sports history are overflowing with such incidents: peak athletes at the top of their game, perfectly coordinated, with seemingly superhuman endurance, strength, and conditioning, who are, on the inside, roiling with disease, one step away from the casket.[37]

When we treat people purely based on those symptoms or signs, we are often operating on the very last stage of a process that has been silently, imperceptibly at work, potentially for years and years.

The Western medical approach is to frantically try to "screen" as many people for as many problems as possible in order to detect the disease earlier and apply a medical intervention (predominately drugs, radiation, and surgery) to restore the positive lab finding back to "normal." So we have blood tests for prostate cancer, mammograms for breast cancer, lipid assays for cholesterol, etc. This is what Western medicine calls "prevention," even though detection and prevention are mutually incompatible terms: We can only detect something we have failed to prevent.

This is why the WHO states so emphatically that being healthy is much more than simply not having symptoms or diseases.

Clinically, the doctor's imperative is to cure disease. Since only a fraction of most of our lives are spent ill, that makes a substantial portion of the physician's realm dealing with "health," even though the physician is not trained to treat health, she is only trained to treat disease. This incongruence represents a serious incompatibility that has real, serious, and documented impacts on American health.

Not only does disease management fail to constitute a health care system because of the problems it misses, but it fails because being healthy involves an entire spectrum of mental, emotional, and physiological performance that exists above the threshold of sickness.

Here's a visual way to look at the multifaceted human condition.

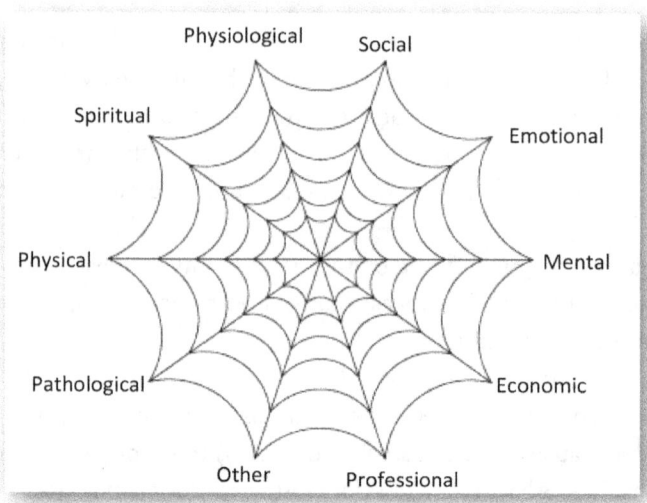

As you can see, a multitude of factors influence the overall picture and each other. In this model, sickness and disease represent just one strand of the web.

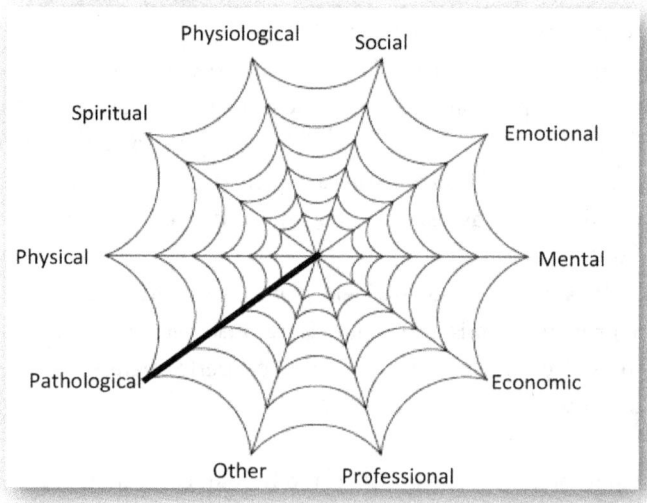

Yet we ask medical doctors to assume responsibility for the management of all strands, essentially trying to turn the web into a simple straight line. It is not the fault of medicine. Doctors are great at treating disease and saving lives. Asking them to be responsible for the staggeringly complex realm of health and well-being is simply beyond their pay grade. Asking medicine and medical health insurance industries to oversee our health inevitably results in health care being reduced to disease care.

Even the prestigious *New England Journal of Medicine* acknowledges these limitations.

"Although the United States pays more for medical care than any other country, problems abound in our health care system. Unsustainable costs, poor outcomes, frequent medical errors, poor patient satisfaction, and worsening health disparities all point to a need for transformative change. Simultaneously, we face widening epidemics of obesity and chronic disease. Cardiovascular disease, cancer, and diabetes now cause 70% of U.S. deaths and account for nearly 75% of health care expenditures. Unfortunately, many modifiable risk factors for chronic diseases are not being addressed adequately. A prevention model, focused on forestalling the development of disease before symptoms or life-threatening events occur, is the best solution to the current crisis...A key feature of U.S. health care is its use of a piecemeal, task-based system that reimburses for "sick visits" aimed at addressing acute conditions or acute exacerbations of chronic conditions. Economic incentives encourage overuse of services by favoring procedural over cognitive tasks (e.g., surgery versus behavior-change counseling) and specialty over primary care. The current model largely ignores subclinical disease unless risk factors are "medicalized" and asymptomatic persons are redefined as "diseased" to facilitate drug treatment..."[38]

Dean Ornish, M.D., who developed the first proven method of reversing heart disease without drugs or surgery, wrote in 1990:

"In America, more money is spent treating heart disease than any other illness—$78 billion annually. Last year, over $7 billion was spent on bypass surgery in this country. If I perform bypass surgery on a patient, the insurance company will pay at least $30,000. If I perform a balloon angioplasty on a patient, the insurance company will pay at least $7,500. If I spend the same amount of time teaching a heart patient about nutrition and stress management techniques, the insurance company will pay no more than $150. If I spend that time teaching a well person to stay healthy, the insurance company will not pay at all. It's not surprising that doctors tend to spend time with what is reimbursed, especially since we do not learn much in medical school about nutrition or how to motivate patients to change their lifestyles. We are not taught skills for coping with stress in our own lives or for teaching these skills to our patients. "[39]

The concept of Pathologization is neither new nor of my own construction. It is a natural consequence of the superimposition of medicine's narrow pathological focus onto the staggeringly multifaceted realm of human health: the Handy Hammer phenomenon. Medicine's limited focus on pathology makes it a valuable (though certainly not exclusive) option for the treatment of illnesses. However, using a hammer to cut sheetrock or paint a house is a poor use of a valuable tool.

Confusing disease care for health care has many consequences. When we substitute disease care (even "preventive" care like screenings) for health care, we promote longevity at the expense of quality of life. We drive up health care costs by promoting and rewarding crisis intervention rather than proactive, supportive, and preventive measures. We fail to successfully deter the progression of illness and disease.

CHAPTER 2

"Preventive" Medicine

What about *preventive* medicine? Isn't that a case of medicine moving toward long-term solutions in health care?

A great deal of energy has been devoted in Western medicine recently to the development of "preventive" medicine. The suggestion here is that medicine is taking a proactive approach to health care, and to a degree this is true. However, it is easy for the public to develop the attitude that preventive medicine somehow represents an authentic movement of medicine into that realm of wellness care. This thinking is a dangerous error, and unfair to medicine. Doctors are simply doing the one thing they do, a little better, and that is a good thing. It is still not health care and should never be mistaken for it.

We are encouraged, nevertheless, to think of prevention as a kind of higher evolution of the medical model and, furthermore, we are encouraged to engage in this model in a very active way. A good example of this public and private engagement is in the realm of cancer.

Cancer is a term that inspires a broad range of feelings, from fear to anger to helplessness, to curiosity and determination. Cancer, as a force, has given rise to a massive infrastructure of cultural and clinical responses, and many of these are highly visible and virtually iconic. We see children wearing colored wrist bracelets, and we are asked to participate in bike rides and walk-a-thons for cancer research. The majority of this energy is focused on what is called cancer "prevention" and research.

In the case of breast cancer, for example, the main thrust of cancer advocacy is toward "prevention" in the form of mammograms. Question: If 100% of all women in the United States between the ages of 40 and 80 had regular mammograms performed, how would this affect U.S. cancer rates?

Answer: not in the slightest degree. Unless you include the iatrogenic factor of applying ionizing radiation to breast tissue in otherwise healthy women, in which case it could be stipulated that the rates would naturally RISE. Mammograms don't prevent cancer; they detect cancer that is already there, and probably has been for a long time.

Magazines and headlines use titles like, "Quest for the Cure," when it comes to breast cancer research and fundraising. The word "cure" is defined by Taber's encyclopedic medical dictionary as a "course of treatment to restore health."[40] "Health," in turn, is defined as "a state of optimum physical and mental well-being, not just the absence of disease or infirmity."[41] This would suggest that individuals seeking a cure would be not merely investigating new treatments for sick people, but seeking to enhance health and discover the *cause* of the disease and address those causal factors so that future generations are less likely to contract the disease.

But most articles feature little to no discussion of things like risk factors, or causes, or prevention, even when they report on the development of screening and treatment options for women with cancer.

Unfortunately, women appear to be acquiring highly inconsistent beliefs about screening and cancer. A recent study of 4,000 women found that 68% believed screening prevents or reduces the risk of *contracting* [my emphasis] breast cancer.[42]

It is unusual, if not outright disingenuous, that the idea of screening is being used synonymously with the idea of prevention. Screening detects disease that has already occurred—hence, has failed to be prevented. Screening is, in a way, the opposite of prevention. It's what we do to determine how much we have failed at prevention. Put another way, screening prevents cancer in the same way that a pregnancy test prevents conception.

And this miscommunication is not limited to breast cancer. Another article recently published in our local paper was entitled, "Colon Cancer—the Number Three Cancer Killer—is Largely Preventable." Yet the article was actually about screening technologies for colon cancer. It contained no real mention or discussion about how to avoid getting colon cancer in the first place, even though we know quite a bit about the causes of colorectal cancers.

It has been stated that certain types of cervical and colorectal cancer can be "prevented" by screening for and removing "precancerous lesions" before they are categorized as cancer. But this is a semantic argument; the surgical removal of a potentially dangerous lesion may be helpful to a patient, but it is not preventive just because the lesion is not called cancer yet.

The American Cancer Society publishes an informational pamphlet called, "Cancer Facts for Women,[43]" which discusses several different types of cancer. This brochure begins each section with a paragraph about the type of cancer, followed by a series of bullet points under the heading, "What You Can Do." Virtually every bullet point offered refers to screening, testing, and medical treatments for women after they already have cancer. References to causes, known dietary contributors to colon cancer, for example, are marginal and not mentioned in the "What You Can Do" sections.

One of the problems with perpetuating the focus on screening and treatment as primary preventive measures is that it gives the public the impression that, if they just follow the recommended guidelines, they will be protected. It promotes a fatalistic attitude toward serious illness, a paradigm which should be subjected to far more scrutiny than it currently is.

Screening may prevent a certain percentage of deaths from cancer, but even this theory has been questioned, as in the recent report in *Lancet* which found no evidence that routine mammography reduces the death rate from breast cancer. A 2006 study from the Cochrane Center in Copenhagen, Sweden, confirmed screening mammograms reduce the absolute risk of dying from breast cancer by 0.05%. Later reviews by the Cochrane Center modified their conclusions. The review includes seven trials that involved 600,000 women in the age range 39 to 74 years who were randomly assigned to receive screening mammograms or not. The studies, which provided the most reliable information, showed that screening did not reduce breast cancer mortality.[44]

Furthermore, the potential risks of mammography are either understated or ignored completely. Many women are unaware that mammograms actually apply radiation, in the form of low dose X-rays, to breast tissue. All X-rays use ionizing radiation, which is a known carcinogen. According to the U.S. Department of Energy, a typical mammogram applies 25 times the radiation of a standard chest x-ray.[45]

Perhaps the best reason to question the way in which cancer screening is promoted is that it does nothing to ensure that our daughters or granddaughters or great-granddaughters will be less likely to contract this disease.

In fact, despite the three billion dollars spent by the American Cancer Society alone since its inception in 1946, worldwide cancer rates reached 12.7 million cases in 2008, and is expected to skyrocket to 21 million by 2030.[46]

One possible reason for the lack of attention to authentic preventive measures in cancer research is that the medical establishment seems to believe that we are "programmed" for cancer, that cancer is a "natural" occurrence. A recent interview with a prominent member of the University of Vermont medical school teaching staff[47] included the statement that cancer is a *normal* part of aging and that nothing can be done to actually prevent it.

Comments like these make it easy to get the impression that, in terms of this issue, medicine has assumed an alarmingly defeatist position.

For example, the following are the primary risk factors identified by the American Cancer Society for women and breast cancer.[48] This is the scientific wisdom gleaned from millions of dollars raised by bike marathons and fundraising walks and pink magnetic ribbons on cars. These are the things women are being instructed to avoid—the things we are telling our daughters to avoid:

Primary Risk Factors for women and breast cancer:

1. Being a woman.
2. Growing older.

Evidently, if we want to prevent cancer in American women, we're going to have to prevent American women, or at least prevent older American women. As a matter of fact, there is a term for this type of reasoning. It is called, "blaming the victim."

And women hoping for words of wisdom about preventing ovarian cancer don't have much to show either. According to the National Ovarian Cancer Coalition,[49] here are the options for reducing the risk of this disease:

1. Go on the pill (despite the increased risk of breast, cervical and liver cancers[50]).
2. Have a tubal ligation (surgical severing of your uterine tubes).
3. Have a hysterectomy (surgical removal of your uterus).
4. Have a "prophylactic oophorectomy" (surgical removal of the ovary).
5. Have children and breastfeed (but start before you're 25).

Predictably, the medical solution is isolated almost exclusively to drugs and surgery. No mention of dietary, environmental, lifestyle, or mental or emotional factors, which may be available to keep women safe. No mention of what a woman can do, outside of drugs and surgery, to prevent this disease if she is over 25 and has not had children yet. She is, presumably, to believe that the significant resources devoted to cancer research, millions of dollars over decades, has failed to discover a single link between diet, weight, exercise, mental health, social conditions, environmental factors such as toxins, pharmaceutical drugs, or quality of life on any other level, and developing cancer. Her choices are to take drugs, surgically disfigure or remove the relevant organ (let's hope they don't transpose this mentality to brain tumors), or start having babies.

It is interesting that this philosophy is not met with more resistance by the American public. Many groups have pointed to the conflict of interest that is inherent in such strategies. It's true that, relative to the simple lifestyle changes and conservative alternative treatments that we already know about, the fantastically expensive high-tech world of treating cancer in people who already have it offers a different level of compensation.

Comedian Chris Rock has a notorious segment he does on this topic in which he shouts, "Ain't never gonna find a cure; ain't no money in the cure—the money's in the medicine!"

But perhaps more germane to the argument is the deeper issue of the unique and limited paradigm of the medical industry, one whose goal is not, nor has ever truly been, the perpetuation of health and wellness, but merely the treatment and care for disease. Understanding that these are two wholly different clinical objectives is critical to understanding the shortfalls of utilizing so exclusively the paradigm of medicine to approach the complex problem of cancer and other degenerative and infectious diseases in our society. To the medical mind, we get sick when we get cancer. To other minds, cancer is a manifestation of a predicating sickness. And this idea of "sickness" is not limited to the individual but expands to encompass the local and global environment with which that individual interacts. Looking for how our diet, our lifestyle, our environment, our air and water quality, our quality of life, and other factors might contribute to getting us sick in the first place hallmarks the mindset behind authentic preventive thinking.

Going to the cause of things has never been the strong suit of medicine, but this is simply because medicine has always been a limited focus specialty field whose realm was essentially saving lives and postponing death. Medicine has always been good at this, never more so than today. But its limited field of vision becomes a liability when the subjects of prevention, wellness, and health arise.

Not until we expand the framework within which we work on the problem of cancer beyond the myopic perspective of the medical paradigm will we even be asking the appropriate questions about how to respond to the problem and safeguard our future generations.

The relationship of lifestyle and environmental factors to cancer incidence has been underreported, underfunded, and under-examined. Recently, the President's Cancer Panel published its findings on environmental cancer risks, in association with the National Cancer Institute, the National Institutes of Health, and the U.S. Department of Health and Human Services.[51] In this report, the Panel stated, "Research on environmental causes of cancer has been limited by low priority and inadequate funding. As a result, the cadre of environmental oncologists is relatively small, and both the consequences of cumulative lifetime exposure to known carcinogens and the interaction of specific environmental contaminants remain largely unstudied."

With the massive amounts of funding, both private and public, that are devoted toward cancer "research," it is certainly somewhat troubling to hear the words "known carcinogens," "environmental contaminants," and "unstudied" used in the same sentence. The Panel later adds that,

"*The prevailing regulatory approach in the United States is reactionary rather than precautionary. That is, instead of taking preventive action when uncertainty exists about the potential harm a chemical or other environmental contaminant may cause, a hazard must be incontrovertibly demonstrated before action to ameliorate it is initiated....Only a few hundred of the more than 80,000 chemicals in the United States have been tested for safety.*"

According to this report, less than one-half of one percent of the potentially carcinogenic chemicals in use in the U.S. have been proven safe. This statistic is shocking. Among the factors influencing this data, the Panel includes "weak laws and regulations, and undue industry influence," which means that the corporations that are profiting from the use of these potentially deadly chemicals are currently able to suppress regulatory control over their use.

The process of identifying and eliminating environmental causes of cancer has a massive flaw. Not only does it fail to generate much capital, but it robs profit from the corporations and industries that subsist on providing technologies and services for the detection and treatment of the disease. Financially speaking, it is a lose-lose situation. This results in what the Panel calls a "lack of will to identify and remove hazards." At worst, you have a situation as occurred in the case of the toxic chemical bisphenol A, or BPA, used in products like baby bottles and food and beverage can liners.

The report adds:

*"Extensive research has linked BPA to breast cancer, obesity, diabetes, and other serious medical problems. The Center for the Evaluation of Risks to Human Reproduction concluded in 2008 that there is "...some concern for effects on the brain, behavior, and prostate gland in fetuses, infants and children at current human exposures to bisphenol A. Yet in 2008, the FDA ruled the BPA is safe even for infants, based on **selected studies** [my emphasis], some of which were **industry-sponsored**, and what is alleged to have been undue influence by industry lobbyists..."*

Included in the 168-page document as implicated carcinogenic contaminants are:

- Contaminants from industrial and manufacturing sources including
  o Polyhalogenated biphenyls
  o Asbestos
  o Chromium (used in the tanning industry)
  o Percholorethylene and trichloroethylene (PCE and TCE, used in dry cleaning)
  o Air pollution
  o Mercury
  o Formaldehyde
  o BPA
  o Phthalates
  o Nanotechnology
- Contaminants from agricultural sources
  o Pesticides
  o Herbicides
  o Fertilizers
  o Veterinary pharmaceuticals

Imagine a road winding through high, steep cliffs. In one section, there is a steep downgrade followed suddenly by a severely sharp curve bordered by a 100-foot sheer drop to jagged rocks below. Chronically poor road conditions and the lack of any railing on the road contribute to a high rate of accidents on this section of road. Now imagine that all of the vast resources of the residents of the area are poured into improved ambulance services for the crash victims, enhanced trauma care at the local hospitals, and the latest in emergency room diagnostic devices. The resources at the bottom of the cliff are vast, and the individuals and corporations that supply them are lauded. Little energy is devoted to preventing the crashes in the first place.

The assumption is that the crashes must be inevitable and the "solution" is defined by reducing the number of fatalities. A small faction of residents advocate for the installation of better guardrails, road signs warning of the upcoming hazard, and improved automobile safety design. Obviously these are not mutually exclusive endeavors, but if one is to be pursued at the expense of the other, who in their right mind would choose the ambulance and trauma care over the safety and preventive measures?

This is not to indict the medical establishment, but it is meant to hold them, and all of us, to a higher standard. That standard includes being honest and accurate when we use terms like "cure" and "prevention." Treatment is not cure. Screening is certainly not prevention. It means being more straightforward about what screening and treatment represent: damage control. It means acknowledging that too few resources are going into finding practical ways to safeguard our posterity from ever getting these diseases, and too little of the conversation is focusing on this objective. It means acknowledging that, as bad as it sounds, there are people in this world who stand to lose a lot of money if an actual cause-cure relationship is discovered. This should make us very skeptical toward the propagation of fatalistic ideologies and summary dismissals of authentic prevention of disease.

Treating people who have cancer is a noble thing. But we should hold ourselves to a much higher standard when we start talking about "cures" and "prevention," because this concerns not only our current generation, but also our progeny. What will our legacy be?

What would cancer research look like if we held ourselves to these standards? The paradigm would focus on establishing long-term (multi-generational) solutions that are pro-active, not just preventive. This means understanding and acknowledging the difference between enhancing health and preventing disease. It means devoting resources into understanding both better, rather than focusing mainly on expensive detection methods and risky treatments. It would mean that cancer research would earnestly investigate known vectors for cancer and known methods for preventing and treating it, even if those methods are alternative, holistic, natural; namely, not profit-making to the medical or pharmaceutical industries. It would mean that the public education campaigns would focus on these vectors; telling us what we can really do to avoid cancer: what to eat, what to avoid, what traditional as well as alternative therapies are worth looking into.

Some researchers believe that women can reduce their risk of contracting breast cancer by as much as 75%[52] simply by introducing dietary and lifestyle changes, such as:

- Consuming fresh, organic fruits, vegetables, and whole grains
- Adding elements such as healthy omega-3 fatty acids, green tea, coenzyme Q, sea vegetables, and various vitamins and minerals
- Reducing red meat consumption, smoking, and dietary and environmental toxins
- Increasing physical activity

And of course it has been shown that natural therapies like chiropractic care and acupuncture can boost the immune system significantly.[53 54 55 56 57 58 59 60 61]

More importantly, this discussion would bring us to the point where we could see the limitations of the prevention paradigm itself. We would encounter an opportunity to look beyond simply avoiding cancer and would expand into an exploration of how to perpetuate and enhance human health and the actualization of our potential on all levels, physical, emotional, and spiritual.

What would a cancer awareness month look like if we held ourselves to these standards? I think our grandchildren are dying to know.

So, while the apex of long-range thinking in medicine is "preventive medicine," it still describes a significant gap between the promise of health care and the limitations of the medical model to provide it. In fact, it could be stated that there is no such thing as preventive medical care. I submit the following evidence:

A typical "checkup" visit to the doctor is, after all, "checking" on only one thing—evidence of disease or impending disease. As a 50-year-old man, I am encouraged to get checked regularly by a physician. Recently, I thought I would see what the M.D.s had to say about my health. I was checked for blood pressure problems, breathing problems, heart problems, prostate problems, blood problems, etc. There was no assessment of my health other than the evidence of signs of illness (nor was I expecting any). They did find that my cholesterol was a bit high. Yet when I received a bill for the visit, I contacted the office to tell them that my insurance paid for all preventive care.

Here's what I got back from the doctor:

```
        ┌                                                      ┐
                  MATTHEW RUSHFORD
                  1 EAST TERRACE
                  SOUTH BURLINGTON, VT 05403

        └                                              ┘
                                        PAY LAST AMOUNT  ▽
                                        IN THIS COLUMN
```

DATE	PROFESSIONAL SERVICES	CHARGES	CREDITS	BAL. DUE
9/5/08	OC initial visit & ins	103.20	ded	103.20
	Spec & "	6.00	"	109.20

After talking to Cigna personally, I do not
feel this could honestly be billed as a
preventative care service since your
Cholesterol is high. Therefore you are
responsible for this bill.
You should also follow up to have your
Cholesterol treated.

What this doctor is contending is astounding: that even preventive medical care is not truly preventive. If you are found to have indicators for illness, prevention has failed. So I had to pay this bill.

Stay with me here, because I have to admit, I got a little lost for a moment myself. If you go to the doctors for preventive care and they find nothing, there has been no preventive care because there are no clinical findings to show that anything has been prevented or needs preventive treatment. The visit itself has done nothing to prevent anything. If they *find* something, this is also, according to them, not prevention, as the existence of positive clinical signs is evidence of the failure of prevention.

This kind of clumsy and ill-informed navigation of the realms of health and disease is representative of the distant and obtuse relationship between medicine and health, and the limitations of a preventive medical model as a pathway to enhanced health.

That doctor, by the way, told me I needed to get on cholesterol medication immediately. Instead, I went to the bookstore, bought a $12 book on diet and heart health, and in two weeks had my cholesterol down to normal. The nurses in the follow-up visit said they had never seen anything like it. I have no doubt they hadn't.

CHAPTER 3
Unhealthy Health Care

We've seen that the establishment of a system of health care managed exclusively by pathology specialists carries with it intrinsic limitations. The clinical and theoretical parameters of medicine are too restricted to adequately consider and care for the broad, complex realm of human health. Truly proactive, preventive measures, which might enable enhanced quality of life and well-being, are difficult to find in the very narrow space within which allopathy lives. These elements, thus, become neglected, and overall health, by association, does as well.

This incongruence also expresses itself in the form of out-of-control costs.

What would have happened if I had taken my doctor's advice and gone on medication for my cholesterol?

One in four Americans over age 45 is currently doing exactly this.[62] The majority are taking statins like Lipitor, which block the enzyme in your liver that makes cholesterol. Back when I had my "preventive checkup," statins were all the rage. Today, just a few years later, they are making news for a completely different set of reasons. It turns out statins not only don't work so well, their limited benefits come at a hefty price.

The New York Times reported in November 2013:

"Statins are effective for people with known heart disease. But for people who have less than a 20 percent risk of getting heart disease in the next 10 years, statins not only fail to reduce the risk of death, but also fail even to reduce the risk of serious illness. Perhaps more dangerous, statins provide false reassurances that may discourage patients from taking the steps that actually reduce cardiovascular disease. According to the World Health Organization, 80 percent of cardiovascular disease is caused by smoking, lack of exercise, an unhealthy diet, and other lifestyle factors. Statins give the illusion of

protection to many people who would be much better served, for example, by simply walking an extra 10 minutes per day."[63]

There are now over 900 studies that point to the dangers of statins.[64]

This simple commentary on a single medical approach to the significant problem of heart disease speaks to the weak impact on health which results from the incongruence between the medical/pharmaceutical skill set and human well-being.

One obvious problem is that it is very difficult to monetize the simple, natural, low-cost and effective preventive measures that actually promote health and discourage illness. As Dr. Dean Ornish said, insurance won't pay for it. On the other hand, the business of waiting for fires and frantically putting them out has never been better:

Alternative medicine advocate Dr. Joseph Mercola reports:

If you think you're spending a lot on health care now, wait a few years. By 2016, it's expected that health care costs will double to more than $4 trillion! And the 16 cents of every dollar that's now spent on health care is going to rise to nearly 20 cents in the next 10 years.

Just about everyone, from businesses to individuals, is feeling the pinch, and it's no wonder when you consider these outrageous facts about health care costs from the National Coalition on Health Care:

- *In 2007, $2.3 trillion, or $7,600 per person, was spent on health care.*
- *Health care spending is 4.3 times the amount spent on national defense.*
- *Total health care spending represented 16 percent of the gross domestic product (GDP), and is expected to increase to 20 percent by 2016.*
- *For comparison, health care spending accounted for 10.9 percent of the GDP in Switzerland, 10.7 percent in Germany, 9.7 percent in Canada, and 9.5 percent in France.*
- *Workers are now paying $1,400 more in premiums annually for family coverage than they did in 2000.*

A review of U.S. healthcare expenses by the Institutes of Medicine[65] has revealed that 30 cents of every dollar spent on medical care is wasted, adding up to $750 billion annually. The report identifies six major areas of waste: unnecessary services, inefficient delivery of care, excess administrative costs, inflated prices, prevention failures, and fraud.

The Institutes of Medicine reports[66] that:

- 50% report that information necessary to their care was not available when needed.
- 1/3 of patients in hospitals are harmed during their stay.
- 1/5 of Medicare patients are re-hospitalized within 30 days.
- 85% of people had not been informed by comparative quality information about their health care.

Medical News Today recently noted that, if each state simply delivered health care at the performance level of the best state, 75,000 lives would be saved every year.[67]

The United States is the only major industrialized nation that fails to provide universal health care coverage. Most other nations also have comprehensive benefit packages with no cost sharing by patients.

Medical debt is the number one cause of bankruptcy in the U.S., and a significant factor in the recent major global economic crisis.[68]

In terms of equity, the U.S. is also last on almost all measures of fairness because we have the greatest discrepancy in terms of quality of care given to the wealthy versus the poor.

Here's just one example from an *Amnesty International* interview from 2009:

Isabel (not her real name), an undocumented immigrant, speaks limited English. She was 27 years old when she went into labor with her first child in 2005. She sought admission at a private hospital close to her home in Memphis, Tennessee. The reception-ist initially turned her away, saying she needed to go to the public hospital, but Isabel insisted her doctor had told her he would meet her there. She told Amnesty International, "I started falling down with pain. In the end they took me in a wheel-chair...I thought I would die, the pain was so bad. They just came in and said, 'Shut up!' A nurse said, 'Everyone can hear you. Shut up or we'll throw you out.' They still had me in a wheelchair the next morning, and I felt the baby coming. I was afraid he would fall on the ground. I was ready to catch him...When my own doctor finally came, I cried. I felt so relieved. If he hadn't come, I would have given birth alone. It's cruel to leave you alone in a hospital.[69]

The New York Times reported on August 12, 2007 that, "this country lags well behind other advanced nations in delivering timely and effective care." The report went on to point out the WHO ranking of nations from 2001 in which the US placed a "dismal

37th." It also mentioned the highly regarded Commonwealth Fund May 2007 report that ranked the U.S. last or next-to-last in most measures of performance, including quality of care and access to care.

Results continue to be a severe problem with the U.S. health care system. According to the *Journal of the American Medical Association*, in a report entitled, "Is U.S. Health Really the Best in the World?"[70], the U.S. ranks last or almost last in terms of the following critical factors:

- infant mortality
- low birth weight percentages
- neonatal mortality
- post-neonatal mortality
- years of potential life lost (excluding external causes)
- life expectancy at one year, 15 years, and 40 years
- age-adjusted mortality
- healthy life expectancy at age 60
- deaths from preventable illnesses
- obesity

That same report disclosed some shocking statistics for iatrogenic (doctor-caused) deaths in the U.S.:

"The health care system also may contribute to poor health through its adverse effects...."

The report goes on to list those effects:

- 12,000 deaths/year from unnecessary surgery 7,000 deaths/year from medication errors in hospitals
- 20,000 deaths/year from other errors in hospitals
- 80,000 deaths/year from nocosomial infections in hospitals
- 106,000 deaths/year from non-error, adverse effects of medications

This is certainly an unusual usage of the term "adverse," in which we actually mean the patient died. That's pretty adverse. In terms of the reliability of these conservative figures, the *JAMA* report stated that, "the poor performance of the United States was recently confirmed by the WHO...Thus, the figures are...robust, and not dependent on the particular measures used."

Robust, again, a sadly ironic term to choose when describing morbidity and mortality of American citizens.

The commentary in this report also cited studies that estimated that "as many as 20%-30% of patients receive contraindicated care."[71]

The costs of adverse drug reactions to society are more than $136 billion annually, greater than the total cost of cardiovascular or diabetic care. Adverse drug reactions cause injuries or death in one out of five hospital patients.[72] As *The New York Times* reported, fatal prescription drug overdoses surpassed car crashes as the leading cause of accidental death in 2007, according to the Department of Health.[73]

One reason there are so many adverse drug events in the U.S. is because so many drugs are used and prescribed. Many patients receive multiple prescriptions at varying strengths, some of which may counteract each other or cause more severe reactions when combined.

Dr. Mercola reports:[74]

"In 2009 there were nearly 3.68 billion prescriptions filled in the U.S. That averages to almost 12 prescriptions for every person in the U.S. The average senior typically fills over 31 prescriptions every year, and even children between the ages of zero and 18 are taking an average of close to four prescriptions annually".[75]

According to the 2011 Health Grades Hospital Quality in America study, the incidence rate of medical harm occurring in the United States is estimated to be ***more than 40,000 harmful and/or lethal errors each and EVERY day.***[76][77]

Put yet another way, our health care system is the third leading cause of death in the United States, after cardiovascular disease and cancer.

Speaking of heart disease and cancer, things don't look too good there either. Heart disease now affects about 80 million Americans and causes more than 860,000 deaths per year, according to the CDC. Cancer is the second leading cause of death and is projected to move to #1 by 2020. Cancer kills one out of every four people in the U.S. and despite all our cancer fundraising and cancer advocacy groups, the number of people with cancer is projected to double in the next 50 years.

In 2012, *Newsweek* reported,

"...Harvey Fineberg, M.D., president of the Institute of Medicine and former dean of the Harvard School of Public Health, had said that between 30 percent and 40 percent of our entire health care expenditure is paying for fraud and unnecessary treatment...A 2010 New England Journal of Medicine study concluded that as many as 25 percent of

all hospitalized patients will experience a preventable medical error, and 100,000 will die annually because of errors..."[78]

To put it into perspective, the figures on preventable deaths represent the equivalent of two jumbo jets filled with men, women, and children, crashing every day of the year, with no survivors.

The question you have to ask yourself is, "If this was an actual airline, would you want to fly it?"

At the heart of our poor results is a fundamental failure to distinguish between health maintenance and disease control and allocate appropriate trained personnel and resources to each. Placing specialists (M.D.s) in charge of the vast and complex world of human health and wellness engenders a blurring of normal and the abnormal, and the increasing tendency to intervene in and disrupt normal body processes.

We over-treat, overmedicate, over-operate, and over-diagnose, and we under-prevent and under-avoid. The U.S represents only 5% of the world's population but we consume over 50% of the world's pharmaceuticals.[79]

Dr. Mercola adds:

The latest study published in Health Affairs revealed that the United States now ranks 49th in the world for both male and female life expectancy, down from 24th in 1999.[80]

*In 1950, the United States was fifth among the leading industrialized nations with respect to female life expectancy at birth, surpassed only by Sweden, Norway, Australia, and the Netherlands. The last available measure of female life expectancy had the United States ranked at forty-sixth in the world. U.S. infants also are in the basement when it comes to mortality rates; according to 2009 data compiled by the World Bank, **the U.S. is 41 places behind other countries in infant mortality.**[81]*

Even though most Americans are unaware of most of these statistics, nevertheless one out of three of us believe that our Health Care system is broken.[82] Streamlining administrative tasks through better use of technology, enforcing greater transparency in order to ensure better horizontal and vertical quality control, and other infrastructural improvements have been suggested to improve results and equity. Yet these logistical changes fail to address the fundamental incongruence between medicine and health. The bottom line is that employing a limited-field clinical specialty such as allopathic medicine as the sole arbiter of the broad, multifaceted, complex realm of human health yields poor results.

PRIMUM NOCERE

One of the principal precepts of medical ethics includes the maxim, "primum non nocere," or, "First, do no harm." The phrase, a version of which is found in the Hippocratic corpus, describes the importance of restraint in the application of medical intervention.

However, the phrase, as it applies to modern medicine, is misleading because it suggests that the application of modern medicine can be anything other than harmful, and this is generally not an accurate representation. The three primary agents of modern medicine—drugs, radiation, and surgery—are all intrinsically harmful, even when they may ultimately result in overall benefit to the patient.

1. DRUGS

America may be the most medicated nation on the planet. According to the U.S. Department of Health and Human Services, at least half of all Americans take at least one prescription drug, with one in six taking three or more medications. We spend over $160 billion per year on drugs. Pharmaceutical intervention is a primary tool of modern medicine.

Drugs are harmful. All drugs have side effects, and most drugs have several side effects. The term "side effect" itself is something of a misrepresentation: what we are actually describing are harmful effects. The definition of a side effect is not just that it is not the intent of the medication, but that it is a deleterious event for the patient. How much more prudence we might exercise in the administration of medicine if we called side effects "harmful effects"! Of course, the term "side effect" has a higher marketing value, as it tends to diminish the significance of these harms.

2. RADIATION

Radiation therapy includes both diagnostic and therapeutic uses of many different types of radiation. MRI's, CT Scans, x-rays, mammograms, and others all use radiation. Radiation is intrinsically harmful, as it exposes the body to focused beams of ionization, one of the few things we know with certainty causes cancer. The harmful effects of radiation are furthermore cumulative, making these harms permanent and irreversible.

3. SURGERY

The harms of surgery are also obvious: In order to perform it, you need to cut into the body. The body must heal the surgeon's cut. It goes without saying that we engage these tools of medicine when we feel that the benefit of the procedure outweighs the harm it inflicts. However, we rarely hear the term, "Harm/Benefit Analysis." Instead we hear "Risk/ Benefit Analysis." And while we should certainly consider both the harm of a procedure as well as the risk of other possible harms, there is a difference between the concept of "risk" and the concept of "harm." The term "risk" implies that the possibility exists for no harm at all. Describing a "Harm/Benefit Analysis," however, more accurately and scientifically describes the process of truly informed decision making in medicine.

Correcting our language when we talk about medicine is an important step in framing the dialogue around medical interventions and the establishment of public health protocols. Failing to identify medicine as intrinsically harmful enables a system in which medical procedures are over-utilized and their harm minimized. A good example is antibiotics. Warnings about excessive prescription of antibiotics have been issued for decades. Etymologists described the impact on humanity as "the worst case scenario" and "the end of the road" more than 20 years ago. Yet pediatricians have made few changes to their habits, decreasing prescriptions by only 20% in that time period. Meanwhile, resistant strains have become so powerful that in 2005, over 18,000 people died from MRSA. That's more than AIDS.[83]

Another good example is the use of painkillers, whose harms are easy to overlook as their benefits are so welcome and immediate. However, not only are we learning about the short and long term "harmful effects" of OTC drugs like acetaminophen and ibuprofen, but the addictive effects of opiate painkillers and the long term harm to the body of that addiction has become a national emergency.

Understanding medicine as inherently harmful is a critical step in reigning in the rampant over-utilization that has affected so many elements of our health care system, and by association, its costs. The health insurance industry does little to help this situation, as its focus on the short term amelioration of the most superficial aspects of health and disease engenders a system that rewards expensive, dangerous interventions and discourages preventive, proactive care.

When we more realistically appreciate the innate harm of medical care, we can make more well-informed decisions about whether and how to utilize it. Sugar-coating the tools of medicine serves no one. The true motto of allopathic medicine should be adjusted to read, "Primum nocere" or "First, the Harm." This is not an insult, but simply embraces the reality that sometimes, in order to help someone, you must hurt them first. Let the world be warned. This terminology shift will help us to choose medical interventions more wisely, and hopefully gain the best that modern medicine has to offer (which is a lot) while avoiding the worst.

Reforming the conversation about our health care system must include:

- Acknowledging the disconnect between health care and disease care.
- Understanding the forces that generated the disconnect.
- Integrating a more complete paradigm of health and wellness into our health care system.
- Dispelling the Pathologization of the Human body, opening up the opportunity to enhance human wellness, performance, and quality of life, naturally.
- Working toward a system in which the highly valuable talents of medicine are judiciously utilized within their realm of specialization, emergency crisis intervention, and integrated into a system that also applies proven strategies for proactive health promotion with minimal intervention and risk.

Part Two
Broken Birth

Introduction
Birth: Pathology or Pathologized?

Remember the Handy Hammer axiom?

"When all you've got is a hammer, everything looks like a nail."

Applied to medicine, the Handy Hammer adage describes the process of Pathologization, in which normal body events and processes, even body parts, are re-framed as abnormal or pathological. It's important to appreciate this phenomenon not as an insidious agenda, but rather simply a natural consequence of the juxtaposition of medicine's limited skill set and training with the vast, complex realm of human physiology and health. Yet Pathologization is not just an intellectual process, it drives clinical protocols and interventions, which impacts patient outcomes in very real ways.

The phenomenon of Pathologization is perhaps most deeply expressed in the processes of pregnancy and childbirth. Childbirth in the U.S. is almost universally medicalized: 95% of women give birth in hospitals, with obstetricians (who are not only medical doctors, but surgical specialists).

Let's take a moment to examine some common assumptions about childbirth:

- Birth was perilous and deadly until it was moved to the hospital.
- Birth is still very dangerous.
- Birth today is best and normal and safest in hospitals.
- Doctors are the best attendants for birth.
- Home birth is more dangerous.

I am going to address all of these notions in the framework of a newly contextualized relationship between our bodies, medicine, and wellness.

As a study of the problems with using medicine to manage normal body processes, birth is a unique and compelling case in point. We invest massively in the institution of hospital birth. Hospitalization related to pregnancy and childbirth costs some US $86 billion a year, the highest hospitalization costs of any area of medicine.[84] Despite this, women in the USA have a greater lifetime risk of dying of pregnancy-related complications than women in 40 other countries. For example, the likelihood of a woman dying in childbirth in the USA is five times greater than in Greece, four times greater than in Germany, and three times greater than in Spain. More than two women die every day in the USA from pregnancy-related causes.[85]

Our perspective on birth has been so deeply informed by medicine that we have difficulty even conceptualizing it outside of a medical setting, specifically, a hospital.

A hospital is defined by Merriam Webster as:

Hospital: an institution where the sick or injured are given medical or surgical care.

Which is a pregnant woman: sick or injured? Technically, pregnancy is a normal body function; in fact, its normalcy is the predication of our existence as a species.

And yet many Americans would be shocked to learn that it is only in America that most women go to doctors for birth.[86] In the rest of the developed world, women give birth in non-medicalized settings, with midwives, and along the way enjoy less intervention and lower rates of complications and mortality. In the five countries with the lowest infant mortality rates in the March of Dimes report—Japan, Singapore, Sweden, Finland, and Norway—midwives were used as the main source of care for 70 percent of the birthing mothers.[87] Even the recent royal birth of Princess Charlotte was attended by midwives, not surgeons.

Nevertheless, nearly all American babies are born in a hospital, and one third of all American pregnancies end in a C-section, which is a major abdominopelvic surgery, despite the fact that the majority of these surgeries lack medical justification. Parents who consider giving birth outside the medical realm are considered reckless and irresponsible. Birth is portrayed in the movies, television, and literature as a medical emergency fraught with peril for the mother and child.

" 'I think this is labor,' she said, looking up. Her hair was loose, a strand caught on her lip. He brushed it back behind her ear. She shook her head as he sat beside her. 'I don't know. I feel strange. This crampy feeling comes and goes...

...'I've been timing them. Five minutes apart. They're strong, and I'm scared.'

He felt an inner surge then; excitement and fear tumbled through him like foam pushed by a wave..."[88]

This excerpt from Kim Edwards' *The Memory Keeper's Daughter* illuminates the unusual and powerful aura of fear that we have come to inject into the process of birth. Why were the husband and wife so afraid? Was there anything abnormal about the labor she was experiencing? No, it was the act of birth itself that was to be feared.

Surely, the media is partially responsible for this perception. Childbirth in the movies and television is more appropriately categorized in the genre of horror than reality. And yet at the same time, this perception coexists with a general belief that birth is also inherently natural. When I give talks to students, community members, or even members of the professional health care community, I always ask how many people think that birth is a normal, natural process. Just about every person in the room will raise their hands. Now, naturally, the next question is, if it is such a normal thing, why do we rush to the hospital like crazy people when it is happening?

Of course, I DO ask this question, and this is where the room generally acquires an awkward, confused silence.

In this next chapter, I'll explore the history of childbirth and how it has come to create such fear.

CHAPTER 4
Primitive Birth

t is a common perception that childbirth was perilous and deadly until it was "saved" by modern medicine. The actual story is far more complex. While we obviously have little hard data on childbirth outcomes in preindustrial times, the evidence we do have suggests a very surprising reality: Childbirth for healthy women living in primitive conditions with no medical care was a short, safe, and relatively easy affair, with little to no danger for mother or child.

The continuum of normal birth has its own genealogy in time and space. We'll begin with birth before doctors, hospitals, and even midwives, at least as we know them today.

What was childbirth like for preindustrial women? Much of what we have is pieced together from oral traditions, early European explorers' accounts, and representations of birth in arts and crafts of pre-modern cultures.

It is, I have found, a popular, though historically questionable, notion that childbirth prior to the advent of modern medicine was fraught with danger and death. It would appear that quite the opposite is the case.

George Engleman (1847-1903) was an American obstetrician whose studies of primitive birth remain the definitive treatise on the subject. His research was featured in medical and surgical journals in his time. In *Labor Among Primitive Peoples*, he writes:

*"Among primitive people, still natural in their habits and living under conditions which favor the healthy development of their physical organization, **labor may be characterized as short and easy, accompanied by few accidents and followed by little or no prostration**; the squaw of the Modoc Indians—a tribe which has been but little affected by the advance of civilization—suffers but **an hour or even less** in the agony*

of childbirth; the Sioux, the Kootenais, and the Santees are somewhat longer in labor, not, however, over two or three hours; two hours being about the average time among the North American Indians. The period of suffering is very much the same among the natives of Africa and of Southern India, the inhabitants of the Antilles and the Caribbees, of the Andaman and the Australian islands, and other savage people.

What **little fear exists as to the occurrence of this event**, which is so much dreaded by many of our delicately constituted ladies, may be judged from the instances of speedy and unexpected delivery so often related by those in contact with the Indians. Dr. Faulkner, who spent some years among the Sioux tribes, tells me that he has known a squaw to go for a pack of wood in mid-winter, have a child while gone, wrap it up, place it on the wood and bring both to the lodge, miles distant, without injury. Dr. Choquette says, that two or three years ago, an Indian party of Flat Heads and Kootenais, men, women, and children, set out for a hunting trip; on a severely cold winter's day, one of the women, allowing the party to proceed, dismounted from her horse, spread an old buffalo robe upon the snow, and gave birth to a child which was immediately followed by the placenta. Having attended to everything as well as the circumstances permitted, she wrapped up the young one in a blanket, mounted her horse, and overtook the party before they had noticed her absence...

...**Accidents rarely occur**; thus, a physician tells me that during a residence of eight years among the Canadian Indians, he knew of no accident, and heard of **no death in childbed**. Another professional brother, who lived four years with the Oregon Indians, was not aware of any irregularity occurring in that time, nor was he ever called upon to perform a more serious operation than the rupture of the membranes....

Commonly **labor is conducted most privately and quietly**; the Indian squaw is wont to steal off into the woods for her confinement. Alone or accompanied by a female relative or friend she leaves the village, as she feels the approach of labor, to seek some retired spot; upon the banks of a stream is the favorite place the world over, the vicinity of water, moving water, if possible, is sought, so that the young mother can bathe herself and her child and return to the village cleansed and purified when all is over. This is true of the Sioux, the Comanches, the Tonkawas, the Nez-Percés, the Apaches, the Cheyennes, and other of our Indian tribes."

These firsthand accounts of childbirth taking place without difficulty, fear, or peril fly in the face of our popular opinion of birth as having been fraught with danger and rescued by medicine. Furthermore, they are consistent across many divergent cultures and regions around the world. Birth was, for reasonably healthy and thriving populations, a normal biological event that typically lasted an hour or two and posed little to no threat to mother or baby. In many cultures, according to Engleman, the mother had or benefitted from little assistance. What would eventually become the role of the midwife was, for many of our ancestors, simply a supportive woman of the tribe who offered emotional and spiritual rather than technical support.

Of birth assistants, Engleman reports:

"With regard to the assistants who aid the parturient woman, there is some difference in the customs of the various races. In many cases she has no help of any kind. As a rule, the assistants, if any, are females, relatives, or neighbors, and the aid they give the sufferer is about the same as that which is too commonly obtained by her more civilized sisters, the world over, often worse than none at all. Occasionally they have professional midwives, whose qualifications depend chiefly upon their age or the number of children they have borne. In case that the patient is a lady of quality, the wife perhaps of a chief, or if the labor proves a very difficult one, the prophet or medicine man is summoned. The physician is mistrusted...."

In an interesting reference to what we now call "Unassisted Childbirth," Engleman describes several cultural precedents:

"In Siam and in Ceram, in parts of Africa and South America, among the Indians of Canada and some of our own—the Tonkawas, the Cheyennes and allied tribes, the Arrapahoes, and the Cattaraugus, there is no class corresponding to our midwives, and the patient has no help whatsoever; but usually relatives and friends aid each other, or there is some assistance rendered by the habitual old woman. This is true of the savage tribes of the vast Russian empire; each village or settlement has an old crone who possesses the power of second sight, and by this gift and other similar means drives away disease; but above all haunts the lying-in room, where she causes much harm to both mother and child by her rude and ill-timed manipulations."

Judith Goldsmith, in her article *Traditional Childbirth,*[89] which appeared in *Mothering* magazine in spring of 1989, offers her depiction of native birth:

"Behind the pile of soft cloths where the woman is sitting, the curtains are drawn. The glow of a fire lights the room. Beside the woman sits another, who is reaching around her shoulders and holding her hand. In back of the woman sits a third, who encircles her waist, massaging her belly. The woman is moaning softly, but mostly she is concentrating,

eyes closed, on the ripples passing regularly through her belly. One of the helping women starts to sing slowly; the rhythms echo those of the birthing woman's body.

The scene could be a tribal village nearly anywhere in the world, in the days before contact with technology. The woman could be Hopi, Balinese, Wolof, or Nepali. The helping women sitting with her could be her mother and grandmother, or an aunt, or perhaps the village midwife.

The first European explorers told wondrous tales of childbirth in other lands. In 1791, a traveler among the Guiana women of South America noted, "When on the march an Indian is taken with labor, she just steps aside, is delivered, wraps up the baby with the afterbirth and runs in haste after the others. Priests who traveled with the first expeditions to North America commented that childbirth among the tribal women was a "short and easy affair": "If a woman was traveling by canoe, she asked to be put ashore, entered the woods alone, returned shortly with the newborn, and resumed her share of the paddling until the end of the journey."

Complications were rare. Adriaen Van der Donck, after visiting North America in 1641, said of the women, "They rarely are sick from childbirth, suffer no inconveniences from the same, nor do any of them die on such occasions."

Recovery was quick. As one writer commented upon visiting the Ila-speakers of northern Zimbabwe, "To those accustomed to the usages of civilization it comes as a shock to see a woman rise up and carry a child, half-an-hour old, back to the house from a shelter in the forest." Likewise, an expedition to South America reported seeing Yamana women "a quarter hour after the event [childbirth] going about their work of rowing, gathering shellfish, lifting loads, as though nothing had happened."

…The Jukun-speaking women of Nigeria continued manual work: cooking, pounding grain, and fetching water from the river or firewood from the bush. Pregnant Navajo women of Arizona would run footraces before sunup when the snow was deep!"

Perhaps the most relevant aspect of tribal birth Goldsmith later reveals:

"…Tribal women did not see childbirth as a time of helplessness, nor did they have their babies "delivered" by specialized practitioners. Tradition taught that the woman herself was the most important agent. Culturally prepared to carry out the birth of her children, the tribal woman maintained a positive and **trusting** [my emphasis] attitude throughout her pregnancy.

In numerous societies, women gave birth with no assistance at all…"

It's important to understand that evolution is a process that takes place over thousands and thousands of years. We have not evolved "modern" anatomical or physiological adaptations. A healthy, well-fed woman in the 21st century has the exact same physiological capability to give birth as the women in these stories. What is different is the environment in which women today, and women throughout history, grow up and live. These environmental factors can indeed impact the experience of childbirth in a radical way.

Because something, clearly, happened.

CHAPTER 5

Corsets, Rickets, and Man-Midwifery: The Real Reasons Birth Became Hazardous

Childbirth may have been "a short and easy affair" for primitive women and their babies, but there is no doubt that, somewhere along the line, this changed dramatically. By at least the 17th century, complications in and around birth had become endemic. Had women's bodies changed that much in the course of a few generations? Biologically, this is a fallacy: Evolution is a process that takes place over millennia, not generations. Women's bodies today are virtually identical to those of women 10,000 years ago.

The biggest change is the environment in which women lived and birthed. Understanding these factors is part of the process of "De-Pathologization": a process of un-demonizing women and their bodies and restoring our fundamental faith in a biological process which, when properly supported and trusted, looks dramatically different and holds an entirely different kind of promise for all involved.

Overall Health

The general health of the majority of Americans in the 1800s was deplorable. It is widely noted that 40% of the American men who volunteered to fight in the Boer War were considered too unhealthy to fight.[90] Improvements in food quality, nutrition, and general health made their greatest advancements in the early 20th century.

"In 1906, a study estimated that two million children were malnourished in the United States. In the early 20th century, doctors and scientists discovered the causes

of pellegra, scurvy, and rickets were deficiencies in niacin, vitamin C and D, respectively... Manufacturers began to enrich flour and milk and other products with vitamins. American diets also improved due to refrigeration, canning, and railroads that made it possible for people to consume milk, fruits, and vegetables year-round, greatly improving their health."[91]

Poor housing conditions were rampant. Backward ideas about health, especially during pregnancy, abounded. These included the widely followed recommendations that a pregnant woman avoid sunlight, fresh air, and exercise![92] Not that, for an urban woman of the 17th century, a stroll through town was anywhere close to hygienic; the degree of public sanitation was such that on many streets it was impossible to navigate on foot from one end to the other without treading in human or animal waste. For instance, in New York City in 1835, more than 10,000 horses dropped about a half million pounds of manure a day on the streets of the city. This, along with human waste, quickly contaminated the local wells of Manhattan. Approximately 3,500 New Yorkers died in the resulting cholera epidemic.[93] One story tells of a Chicago woman at this time who attempted suicide by throwing herself in the local river. She immediately found the water to be so putrid and foul that she abandoned her scheme, swam out, and went back home!

Historical accounts of private and public health conditions prior to the 20th century are voluminous; this is just a brief consideration. The important impact that poor health conditions had on childbirth is obvious and direct: A woman who is unhealthy is more likely to have complications in birth than a healthy woman. Public hygiene and sanitation measures began to take effect in the early and mid 20th century, including the purification of public water supplies. This is widely agreed to have had a major impact on morbidity and mortality, particularly for people living in urban centers.[94]

Women's Rights

Another factor which influenced birth outcomes and which saw dramatic changes in the early 20th century was women's rights. How do women's rights affect birth outcomes?

First, if a woman lacks the agency to self-determine her own pregnancy, then the pregnancy is not on her terms and risk factors rise sharply. It may be difficult in this era of the modern family to imagine the degree to which women's control over their own pregnancies was out of their own hands, but it's worth taking a short trip, not too far back in time....

In *A History of Women's Bodies*, Edward Shorter writes of life for an 18th century woman:

"In our own time, a married woman who dislikes her husband's advances can leave the marriage, and an unmarried woman is usually able to avoid a man's embraces if she so wishes. But today we have the "modern," even "postmodern" family, and things are very different from two hundred years ago, when the traditional husband's "conjugal rights" meant that the married woman could not in fact refuse intercourse...

Put yourself in the shoes of the typical housewife who lived in a small town or village then. Neither she nor anyone else had any idea when the "safe" period for a woman was, and for her, any sexual act could mean pregnancy. She was obliged to sleep with her husband whenever he wanted. And in the luck of the draw, she would become pregnant seven of eight times..."[95]

The subordination of women in this era was complete and unquestioned: "The woman had the status of 'the chief servant of her sons and of the farmhands,' while the man was 'master of his little kingdom,' or *Herr im Hause* as the Germans said."[96] The scope of what Shorter calls "the male unconcern for the welfare of women" at this time is staggering. Even the folk sayings of the time reflected the astonishing hierarchy:

If the cow kicks off, mighty cross.
If the wife kicks off, no big loss.
Got a dead wife? No big deal.
Got a dead horse? How you squeal.[97]

The result of this dehumanization process is that women chronically became pregnant when they were incapable or unprepared for the pregnancy, the birth and/or the baby, by virtue of her current health, workload, or mental state. Often women became pregnant too soon after a prior pregnancy, when their bodies had not recovered. This compounded the risk factors for her pregnancy geometrically, and in ways her primitive ancestors never had to navigate. In order for childbirth to follow its biological blueprint, the information the woman holds about her body's health and readiness for pregnancy must be a factor in the pregnancy itself. She must have some agency in her own reproduction in order for a healthy, normal birth to occur.

Her primitive sisters may have exercised a child spacing of approximately three to five years, but amidst her "perfect storm" of biological ignorance and cultural discontinuity, men had such lack of concern for women and women lacked such self-determinism that often women would become impregnated while still in convalescence from a recent childbirth! One can imagine the disastrous impact on that ensuing pregnancy.

The important thing to recognize is that these complications did not occur because the woman was giving birth—they occurred because the woman was *unwell* and giving birth. Assigning the pathology to the correct source is critical here if we are to honestly assess the intrinsic risk in the birth process. Lack of women's rights is obviously still a major problem in many developing countries. In the U.S., women still lacked the right to vote in 1919, but within 30 years, the 19th amendment and the birth control pill would both be a part of American life.

Rickets

The impact of rickets on birth outcomes in the United States can hardly be exaggerated. Rickets, a softening of bones in children, is caused by a deficiency of Vitamin D. The increase in vitamin deficiencies like rickets paralleled the rise of the industrial society. With industrialism came poor nutrition and less exposure to sunlight. Unfortunately, little was known, at the dawn of the Industrial Revolution, about vitamins, or nutrition itself. The very existence of vitamins was not even discovered until the early 1900s. Parents believed that exposure to cold air caused sickness and kept their babies out of the sun.[98]

The prevalence of rickets in the U.S. into the early 20th century was staggering. Some sources indicate that 95% of American children had rickets by the age of eight months.[99]

Rickets alters normal bone formation; in the case of the pelvis (one of the last bones to ossify), a malformed pelvis almost unilaterally means a more difficult childbirth. The shape of the pelvis determines the shape of the opening through which the fetus will pass. The prevalence of rickets, then, was a major contributing factor to the prevalence of difficult, painful, and hazardous births in the 18th, 19th, and early 20th centuries. The malformed ricketic pelvis made childbirth, for many, torture. It was not representative of normal healthy birth, though it was representative of *typical* birth of the time.

Discovery of the link between vitamin D and rickets in 1935[100] and passage of the Fair Labor Standards Act in 1938 helped to eventually cure rickets and free children from the confinement of inside work which deprived them of the sunlight needed for proper skeletal development.

Corsets

The Victorian corset, or "stay" as it was also called, was a garment composed of a flexible material, fabric or leather, stiffened with boning, called ribs or stays, inserted into sleeves in the fabric.

Historians debate both the prevalence of corset use in America and the impact of the corset on female anatomy. It is widely believed that widespread use of the corset by women in both Europe and the west in the 16th, 17th, and 18th centuries had a dramatic impact on women's anatomy and physiology.

However, Shorter insists this image is inflated:

"According to one historian of the 19th century [Axel Hansen]: In no other age throughout history was...the female body so concealed and disfigured by clothing...A long line of physicians opposed the device including Samuel Thomas Soemmerring, who thought corsets responsible for spinal deformities, tuberculosis, all sorts of internal bleeding, fainting, diarrhea, prolapse, and so on.

Although the corset has been paid endless attention in the history of fashion, two essential points have been missed. (1) Outside of the aristocracy and urban middle classes, very few women ever wore corsets; (2) Whether they wore them does not much matter from the viewpoint of their health because the corset was essentially innocuous."[101]

Shorter's point of view is certainly the minority. Sociologist Leigh Summers refers to the multitude of fashion plates, advertisements, and public discussion over the "20-inch waist" as evidence that supports the belief that use of the corset was prevalent in the latter half of the 19th century across classes, and they were worn tight and worn young (a popular saying at the time was that a woman's waist shouldn't measure more in inches than her age of marriage in years. Most women married around the age of 21).

Oscar Wilde, as editor of *Woman's World,* said that the corset had "by slow degrees deformed the figure," causing a woman's body to have "lost its elasticity and ceased to develop according to the laws of nature"

In her book *Pushed,* Jennifer Block discusses Summers' conclusions:

"The corset exerted up to 80 pounds of pressure per cubic inch, cramping circulation, often causing swelling in the legs and a visible pulse at the temples. Pelvic floors deteriorated, uteri prolapsed, and miscarriages (some deliberate) ensued. The corset even created its own syndrome, chlorosis, a term that referred to the triad of menstrual cessation, shortness of breath, and fainting spells, a severe form of anemia. This condition, originally attributed to the fragile female constitution, mysteriously disappeared with the arrival of the drop-waist flapper dress...."

Block also refers to Alice B. Stockham, one of the first female doctors in the U.S., who found a connection between the corset and reproductive issues. "The corset, more than any other one thing, is responsible for women being the victim of disease and doctors," Stockham wrote in her book, *Tokology,* in 1883.

Beginning with their origination as padded, quilted, unboned French waistcoats in the mid 1700s, corsets experienced an almost perpetual escalation in rigidity and constriction. Padding was replaced by boning, the baleen of whales being a common element. By the 1850s, whale bone was replaced by steel and metal eyelets made extremely tight lacing possible.

And to the degree that corsets were utilized, they clearly exerted a devastating effect on the anatomy and physiology of any woman hoping to give birth.

Corsets fell out of fashion in the 1920s, replaced by girdles and elastic brassieres. Interestingly, birth outcomes began to improve at this point in American history. A spike in mortality appears around 1910-1920, when childbirth was being moved to the hospital. It took 30 years or more for hospital birth to catch up to the rate of decline that was being seen in home births.

Lithotomy Position

Of all the issues around modern birth practices that I discuss in my presentations, it is the history and anatomy and physiology of the lithotomy position that generates the most emotional responses from the audience.

Prior to the 16th century, women birthed in a variety of positions. Traditional birthing accessories have included everything from straps of cordage suspended from a ceiling or tree to the Dutch birthing stool used in Babylonia over 4,000 years ago and still in use today.[102]

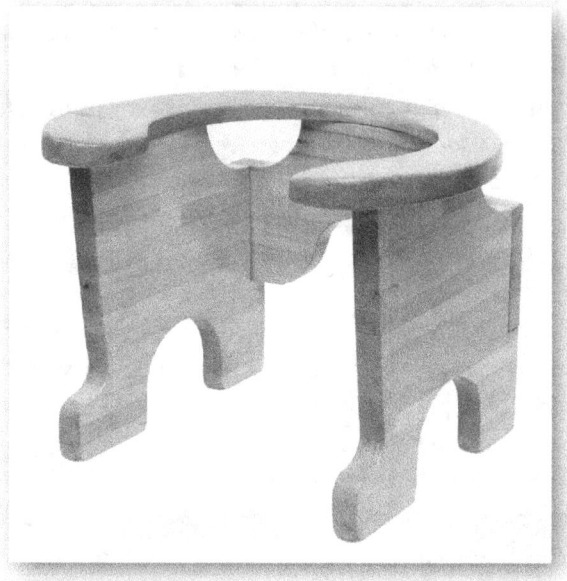

One constant remained unchanged and universal, across cultures, continents, and centuries, and indeed remains true today even in the age of overwhelming medicalization of birth: A woman, left to her own devices and following the natural cues of her body, will almost always birth in an upright position. The reason for this is obvious, simply that it is intuitive to assume a position that capitalizes on the factors of gravity and leverage when confronted with the substantial physical challenge of delivering an eight pound human through an opening that is normally less than four inches in diameter.

In all of recorded human history, this simple, self-evident reality remained unchanged, until the end of the 16th century, when the male-dominated barber surgeons of Europe began to infiltrate the field of childbirth and compete with the traditional birth attendant, the midwife.[103] The barber-surgeons tended to be called in to the more extreme cases in which the lives of the mother and/or baby was in danger; hence, they tended to utilize more aggressive interventions, like extraction techniques. These interventions are of course more difficult to perform when the woman is in her natural squatting position (not to mention the unacceptably inferior physical position it requires the male attendant to assume). This fact naturally led the medical men to advocate for birthing positions and beds which would better facilitate their heroic interventions.[104]

Two men would ultimately advance this cause beyond, perhaps, the wildest expectations of those early barber-surgeons. The first was French physician Francois Mauriceau (1637-1709). Mauriceau also has the dubious distinction of being one of the earliest physicians to attempt to re-frame the normal process of pregnancy as inherently pathological. He actually referred to pregnancy as a "tumor of the belly" caused by the fetus. Mauriceau in 1668 wrote *The Diseases of Women with Child and In Child-Bed*, in which he recommended all women be placed in a "reclining" position for birth.[105] How widely or quickly these recommendations would have been adopted would soon be answered by the second man to advance the cause of the lithotomic position, the King of France.

It is now commonly known that King Louis XIV of France was a man of unusual, some would say perverted, sexual fetishes. One of these fetishes involved his gaining sexual satisfaction from watching women giving birth. Unfortunately, the traditional upright position for birth made satisfying this caprice quite prohibitive. Louis demanded that women assume a supine position for birth so that he may see their genitals as they performed the act. This rather unusual inclination is widely credited with advancing the more universal adoption of the lithotomic position in childbirth.[106]

NURSERY RHYMES AS CULTURAL MEMORIES

This movement of birth towards universal supination, away from the way women had brought forth life from the earliest beginnings of humanity, represents a major benchmark in the evolution of the act of bearing children. As humans, we tend to register these seminal moments in our collective history by embedding them in the infrastructure of our common language, song, and literature as archetypes. Joseph Campbell said that "myths are public dreams, dreams are private myths," and persistent myths (in the form of songs, stories, poems, or images) are like recurring dreams.

They persist because they say something important about our history and our nature. These archetypes are hidden forms, clues to the collective unconscious, signposts which help us navigate temporally and generationally in the context of the larger social and spiritual continuum. They are totems which appear spontaneously in popular culture, media, art, music, etc.—necessarily obtuse and indirect, coded expressions of a universal anthropological compass. Nursery rhymes are rife with archetypes, as they are designed to speak to the young, unformed mind, still open to the language of imagination and ciphers. In The Time Falling Bodies Take to Light, historian William Irwin Thompson suggests that Humpty Dumpty is a rhyme about the formation of the universe and the Fall of Man into consciousness and duality.[107]

Frere Jacques is a song that children sing about a monk that was brought into the court of Louis XIV to demonstrate his supine position for gallstone surgery.[108] The song is believed by some to be based on Frere Jacques Beaulieu, who was a lithotomist (a surgeon who specialized in removing gallstones) brought into the French royal court in the mid 17th century.[109] This was at a time when, by order of the king, the births were to be conducted in the "lithotomy" (supine, or laying on one's back) position, rather than the position in which women had given birth in virtually all of recorded prior history, in the upright position, some variation of a squat.

The royal edict, as often is the case, quickly became adopted as de rigueur of the times, and the lithotomy position was adopted by women throughout Europe as the proper way to give birth. However, the popularity of this new tradition did not change the fact that it represented a fracture in the cultural and spiritual continuum of this important ritual, or the fact that the new practice exerted an oppressive force on laboring women, slowing their labors, choking their fetuses, and strangling their birth muscles, jeopardizing their children and themselves.

Frere Jacques, FrereJacques,
Dormez-vous? Dormez-vous?
Sonnez les matines! Sonnez les matines!
Ding, daing, dong. Ding, daing, dong.

Not surprisingly, the song is nothing more than a question:

Frere-Jacques,
Are you sleeping?
The bells are ringing...

As if to say, "Why are you laying down? Are you asleep, even though the bells ring?" Perhaps the question is meant for the millions of women who continued to give birth on their backs, against every instinct in their bodies, minds, and spirits. Are you sleeping? What other reason would you have to be in such a posture? The bells are ringing. Wake up!

The use of this position was naturally more convenient to any practitioner assisting the laboring mother. As both the utilization and scope of medical intervention grew, so did the use of the lithotomic position.

Interestingly, the U.S. adopted an even more radical and counter-intuitive position, that of the woman lying flat on their back. European practices varied at this time, but most favored some sort of reclining or side posture; none had the woman flat on her back.

Many feminists and natural birth advocates will characterize the adoption of the lithotomy position as a symbol of the male-dominated medical realm's war against women and women's rights.

Robbie Davis Floyd discusses its symbolic significance:

"This lithotomy position completes the process of symbolic inversion that has been in motion since the woman was put into that "backwards" hospital gown. Now we have her normal bodily patterns of relating to the world quite literally turned upside down: her buttocks at the table's edge, her legs widespread in the air, her vagina totally exposed. As the ultimate symbolic inversion, it is ritually appropriate that this position be reserved for the peak transformational moments of the initiation experience: the birth itself."[110]

At the same time, we can see that, in the case of surgeons like Mauriceau, advancement of the new procedure was driven, at least in part, by the simple logistical needs of the new and evolving field of medical obstetrics, not to mention in most cases an apparently earnest desire to bring ease and comfort to the patient. This field, a child of the scientific revolution, saw its growth paralleled (and, many historians argue, fed) by the industrial revolution. One casualty of industrialization was the overall health of the general population, particularly its female citizens. Poorer health meant a greater need for emergency intervention. Enter the new physician, riding the coattails of the new science.

A greater supply of sick people led to a greater demand for surgeons, which led to a greater demand for those procedures and implements, which facilitate emergency obstetrical intervention. This is not to say that the practices of the obstetric field were not influenced by the intrinsic paradigm of its male-dominated orientation (the word "obstetrics" comes, after all, from the root meaning, "to stand in front of") but simply to add an additional element to the timeline of obstetrical interventions. The adoption of the supine position for birth was as much an invention of practicality as it was an expression of sexual hierarchy.

Nevertheless, the development of such procedures as the use of the lithotomic position reflected the overall erosion of a woman's sense of self-determinism in birth. In fact, when we examine the final product of this longer evolutionary process, one that originates with essentially safe and easy primitive birth and reaches its apex in the ultra-medically managed birth-as-pathology model, with the mother to be strapped to a table on her back, drugged senseless and literally sliced open, the baby ripped from her with cold, alien "iron fingers" while she screams in agony, it's hardly hyperbolic to suggest that the sum total of the obstetric influence has been in no small way deleterious to the empowerment of women.

By the early 20th century, the lithotomic position was unquestioned as the only appropriate way to give birth, at least in a medical setting. It is interesting to note how short our collective historic memory is when you mention the tradition of giving birth on one's back. In my classes, the general initial sentiment is that this is a wholly normal and efficient manner to give birth. Furthermore, the same general assumption is made of this procedure as virtually every other medical procedure, namely that the transition (as it is also generally vaguely recognized that at some point in our distant history women must NOT have given birth like this as a rule) occurred with the strength of science and for the proven benefit of the patient. Of course, neither was the case. The transition occurred purely for the convenience of the physician, or in the case of one of its proponents, the titillation of its audience. As for the patient, it would be difficult to imagine a less conducive position for giving birth.

Roberto Caldeyro-Barcia, past president of the International Federation of Obstetricians and Gynecologists, states unequivocally,

"Except for being hanged by the feet, the supine position is the worst conceivable position for labor and delivery."[111]

Floyd describes the physiological impact of the lithotomic position:

- The weight of the woman's body and baby is focused on the tailbone, which pushes it forward and narrows the opening through which the baby must pass. This makes labor longer and more difficult.

- The position compresses all the major blood vessels and nerves of the abdomen and pelvis, which cuts off blood and nerve supply to the baby, increasing the chances for fetal distress. Several studies showed a 91% DECREASE in oxygen saturation in the fetus.
- It also causes weaker and less frequent contractions.
- Pushing is harder because of going against gravity, increasing risk of forced extraction with forceps, vacuum or manual techniques.

Asking women to give birth on their backs violates every innate impulse the woman has, yet two things nevertheless occurred: 1) women agreed (what choice did they have?); and 2) women somehow still managed to give birth, albeit with significant increase in complications, pain, and death.

Taken together, the cumulative impact of poor hygiene, sanitation, nutrition, physical health and activity, and diabolical fashion and medical trends, had an impact on women and birth that was both devastating and unprecedented. Women, in general, and particularly those of the middle and lower classes (representing the large majority) were overworked, undernourished, and physically disfigured by disease, malnutrition, abuse, and corsets. They lived in abominable sanitary conditions and had limited access to healthy physical elements such as fresh air, sunshine, and exercise. They had no agency to self-determine their own reproduction based on their own knowledge of safety and health. Virtually every aspect of what we now recognize as the essential elements of healthy pre-natal conditions were either deeply deficient or wholly absent.

The impact on the act of childbirth was direct, pandemic, and inescapable. Childbirth became, for many, a tortuous act fraught with peril, both to mother and child. So widespread were labor complications that a common obstetric intervention in cases of protracted labor was to insert instruments into the vagina to crush its skull and then remove the fetus' body piece by piece in an effort to at least save the mother's life.[112] This was, in fact, the primary intervention of obstetricians prior to the 18th century.

In order to understand the desperation that birth caregivers felt, one must understand these unusual and drastic conditions that birth attendants experienced and the altered birth outcomes they engendered. Prior to the discovery of relatively safe anesthesia in the late 1800s, attendants were left to only watch and comfort both surgical and obstetric patients who encountered massive and often shock-inducing pain. The fact that these complications, particularly to the degree that they occurred in the population, were not in any way representative of the inherent biological process of childbirth seems to have never been considered, even after those conditions that prompted the radical obstetric interventions were ameliorated. With what we have seen in modern times, with the attribution of chronic illnesses to unsolvable, obscure congenital forces even as evidence of environmental and behavioral causes piles up, this is hardly shocking.

The very man who is credited with the development of both ether and chloroform for use in midwifery, James Simpson Young, was allegedly powerfully motivated by an experience he had in his early training in which he witnessed a mastectomy performed on a patient without anesthesia. Joseph DeLee, whom we'll meet soon, was clearly affected by the calamitous birth experiences he saw at the Chicago Lying-In Hospital.[113]

Here in Vermont, you can drive 10 or 15 minutes in nearly any direction and find a small town graveyard filled with gravestones from this era. Many of the plain granite markers bear the weather-worn names of young mothers and babies who died in childbirth. The idea that childbirth was a life-threatening experience that was "saved" by doctors and hospitals is powerfully influenced by our cultural memory of this dramatic period of our history, and one of the most pervasive and fallacious myths of modern history.

The growing frequency of childbirth complications combined with the advent of the medical hospital in the 18th century[114] created a perfect storm for childbirth problems. More and more women found themselves birthing in hospital environments. However, without modern understanding of the epidemiology of disease and microbes, hospitals were not safe environments for women in childbirth. They were deathtraps. At the center of this macabre portrait is the scourge of childbed fever.

CHAPTER 6
Ignaz Semmelweis: A Tale of Two Clinics

Childbed fever was indeed a very real epidemic, and it was neither limited to the U.S. nor to the 19th and 20th century. In some European hospitals in the 16th and 17th century, more than 50% of birthing women died of the disease.[115] In the United States as late as 1920, as many as 40% of all maternal deaths were attributed to it[116]; some sources say the number is closer to half.[117] "A woman could be delivered on Monday, happy and well with her newborn baby on Tuesday, feverish and ill by Wednesday evening, delirious and in agony with peritonitis on Thursday, and dead on Friday or Saturday."[118] Childbed fever, or puerperal sepsis, is also at the center of a fascinating and deeply symbolic chapter in medical history.

At the center of this chapter is a physician named Ignaz Semmelweis. In Semmelweis' Germany, childbed fever was a deadly enigma of 19th century European birth clinics. As to the cause of childbed fever, the medical paradigm of the time had some unusual explanations. Since there was no awareness of microorganisms or infectious disease, puerperal sepsis was attributed to such ambiguous causes as crowdedness, poor ventilation, beginning lactation, and changes in the weather.

In reality, women were dying of puerperal sepsis mainly because of the place in which they were giving birth: hospitals.

Historian Edward Shorter, whose *A History of Women's Bodies* is anything but biased toward midwifery care, writes:

"No more septic environment can be imagined than that of the maternity hospital before the advent of antisepsis late in the 19th century. Here is the Paris Hotel Dieu in 1788. "One judges the dirtiness of a ward by its odor," Jacques-René Tenon advised his readers. "To really get an idea of what smell is, one should turn up here in the morning, at wound-dressing time." Of course, this was inevitable, he said, when they were obliged to place

the huge beds every-which way, "with little alleys and dim passageways among them, where the walls are covered with spittle, the floor covered by the filth that drains from the mattresses and from the commodes when they're emptied, as well as with the pus and blood that pours down from wounds or bloodlettings." Tenon went on to explain that infected and healthy mothers were placed side by side in the same bed, in the same stinking room as the terminal venereal-disease cases, in wards right on top of the hospital's morgue. And the hospital's laundry was heaped in a chest at the end of the delivery room, "fermenting there and increasing the corruption."[119]

But until Pasteur provided a plausible mechanism for microbiological contagion, the causes of childbed fever remained esoteric.

Enter Ignaz Semmelweis.[120] In July 1846, as the U.S.-Mexican war was in its early stages, Semmelweis became the house officer of the First Obstetrical Clinic of the university's teaching institution, The Vienna General Hospital (Wien Allgemeines Krankenhaus). His most urgent problem to solve was the high maternal and neonatal mortality rates due to puerperal fever—over 13%. Interestingly, the Second Obstetrical Clinic had a mortality rate of only two percent. What was the difference between the First Obstetrical Clinic of the Vienna General Hospital and the Second Obstetrical Clinic of the Vienna General Hospital? Absolutely nothing. The entire staff was perplexed by the contrast, as no clear explanation was apparent. This is because the entire staff ignored one difference that indeed existed between the two clinics, a difference that you may have guessed if you have been reading carefully: While the First Clinic was a teaching service for medical students, the Second Clinic was run by midwives.

Semmelweis stumbled upon an answer to the riddle of puerperal fever when his friend, Jakob Kolletschka (1803-1847), professor of forensic medicine at Vienna, died unexpectedly. Kolletschka's finger had been accidentally punctured during a post-mortem examination, and his own autopsy revealed a disease process that reminded Semmelweis of puerperal fever.

In a moment of classic scientific revelation, Semmelweis made the critical association between puerperal fever and cadaveric contamination. He concluded that he and the students were unwittingly transporting some kind of infecting particles from the autopsy room to the examination room.

Now here the casual student of medical history reads on to discover the revolutionary system of hand sanitation that Semmelweis devised that cured puerperal fever. He proposed that physicians wash their hands in a chlorinated lime solution before doing pelvic exams.

But why, when the directors originally discovered the radical incongruence between the midwife-run clinic and the doctor-run clinic, did they not simply try to duplicate the methods of the midwife clinic? That would seem the simplest, most straightforward way to correct a horrible scourge that was killing hundreds and thousands of women and children year after year after year. This did not happen.

Nevertheless, Semmelveis' discovery was monumental.

But it was not well-received.

In Semmelweis' own clinic, he encountered strong resistance, especially from the medical students and staff. Eventually, he managed to institute a hand washing protocol and in barely **one month** the mortality from puerperal fever declined in his clinic from 12.24 percent to 2.38 percent.

However, this chapter of medical history hasn't even begun to get interesting.

Despite continued results that Semmelweis documented fastidiously, the medical community was somehow unmoved and generally unsupportive of his discovery. Even the director of his clinic was critical of his protocols. Although Semmelweis statistically proved his eradication of puerperal fever, a proposal for an official commission to investigate the results was inexplicably denied by the Ministry of Education. But things were just starting to go south for our friend Ignaz.

His boss, angered that the positive results Semmelweis had achieved represented an indictment of his own failure to support them, refused to reappoint Semmelweis. He managed to acquire an unpaid position at the clinic, but was fired shortly thereafter. When he then applied for a job at the midwife clinic, he was rejected.

In 1850, after having delivered a series of lectures on his findings to the Association of Physicians in Vienna, he nevertheless encountered so little support that he was forced to move suddenly to Pest, Hungary. He was appointed head of the maternity ward at the hospital, which coincidentally, was reeling from an epidemic of—you guessed it—puerperal fever. Semmelweis took charge of the department and enacted his prophylactic measures and soon reduced the mortality rate to a mere 0.85 percent. This occurred at a time when mortality in Prague and Vienna was still between 10 and 15 percent.

In 1861, Semmelweis finally published his momentous discovery in book form, *Die Ätiologie, der Begriff und die Prophylaxis des Kindbettfiebers*. Again, astonishingly, his findings were met with unfavorable reviews. It was now 14 years since Semmelweis had cured childbed fever, and the medical community continued to reject his work. He lashed out with a series of open letters to the obstetrical community, whom he calls "irresponsible murderers." This, predictably, did little to help his standing among his peers.

The same year Semmelweis' spirit was finally broken. He knew he had discovered a cure, but could only stand by and watch as thousands of mothers and babies died. Ignaz Semmelweis went, quite literally, mad. He was committed to an asylum in July, 1865. He died only two weeks later.

Before his death, he wrote,

"When I look back upon the past, I can only dispel the sadness which falls upon me by gazing into that happy future when the infection will be banished...The conviction that such a time must inevitably sooner or later arrive will cheer my dying hour."

Sadly, many years went by before his cure was honestly considered and ultimately applied. Into the 1920s, puerperal sepsis remained a significant clinical entity. Pause a moment to take in the enormity of this delay. In four decades—less time than it took medicine to accept and adopt Semmelweis' *proven, documented, and tested* cure—the field of aviation progressed from the Wright brothers' 59 second flight to supersonic air travel. And although Semmelweis' "conviction" that science would ultimately prove the rightness of his mission was correct, though staggeringly protracted, the treatment he received at the hands of his peers will also become historic.

The "Semmelweis Reflex" was dubbed by Timothy Leary in *The Game of Life*:

The Semmelweis Reflex

"Mob behavior found among primates and larval hominids on undeveloped planets, in which a discovery of important scientific fact is punished rather than rewarded. Named after Dr. Ignaz Semmelweis, who discovered the cause of puerperal fever, a now-obsolete disease which, in Semmelweis's primitive era, killed a vast number of women in childbirth every year. Semmelweis was fired from his hospital, expelled from his medical society, denounced and ridiculed widely, reduced to abject poverty and finally was beaten to death in a madhouse."

In case you think the Semmelweis Reflex is an antiquated vestige of 17th century thinking, consider Dr. Sherwin Nuland, respected author of medical nonfiction books such as *How We Die*.

In *Doctors: The Biography of Medicine*, Nuland excoriates Semmelweis for being "too stubborn"[121] and "self-righteous."[122] He blames Semmelweis' failure to present his findings in an appropriately nonthreatening tone for the delay in the acceptance of his ideas. He places Semmelweis at fault for failing to save "the many lives that were tragically lost because of his obdurate posture."[123] He accuses Semmelweis of "conceit" and "grandiosity that would eventually sweep him to his destruction." This rather ruthless character assassination contradicts the image we have that medicine is a field wholly subservient to the ethic of the scientific method, for Semmelweis lacked no data or evidence to support his claims.

The resistance to his reform, even Nuland admits, was pure self-interest:

"It must have been difficult for the aging Klein [Johann Klein, the chief of obstetrics at the Vienna Clinic] to contemplate his own role in the carnage. Accepting the Semmelweis doctrine would have forced him not only to acknowledge the validity of his opponents' logical method of objective reasoning, but also to admit his unknowing complicity...in the deaths of thousands of young women..."[124]

Klein instead responded by firing Semmelweis.

The Semmelweis Reflex, thus, is not a historical footnote, but a living document, a cautionary tale about the conflicting forces of professional self-interest and scientific truth.

Oliver Wendell Holmes, after all, also proposed that puerperal fever was a contagion dispersed by physicians. In fact, his proposal predates Semmelweis by several years. And while Holmes lost neither his position nor his mind in the process, his theories were soundly repudiated by his contemporaries,[125][126][127] some of whom suggested that the agent of puerperal fever was the nervous, mentally fragile woman herself.[128]

The fatal flaw of Semmelweis' theory is that it required doctors to consider a paradigm of health and disease that was beyond the currently accepted belief system. Not until Pasteur and Lister framed the conversation in the context of microorganisms and the pathology of unseen infectious agents could the medical scientific community consider the truth of Semmelweis' findings. Unfortunately, this failure resulted in the unnecessary loss of thousands of innocent lives. We face the same kind of imperative to execute a quantum leap in our perception of health and disease.

But what is perhaps most interesting is our reluctance, throughout history, to solve the perpetual problems of mixing medicine with childbirth by simply seeking to reproduce the methods that are utilized by the practitioners who have consistently achieved the best results in birth: the midwives. After all, the mortality rate at the Second Clinic of Vienna was one-tenth that of the First.[129] In fact, every time the First

Clinic closed down, the epidemic would stop![130] To me, the moral of the story is that we should never underestimate our collective ability to ignore blatant truths that conflict with our current world views.

It's worth pointing out here that midwives do not achieve superior results because they possess esoteric and secret technology or learning. Midwives achieve greater success because they operate on a different paradigm. This paradigm simply states that childbirth is a natural phenomenon and not a disease—pregnancy and birth are "non-pathologized." It states that women should be empowered and supported in birth, not "treated" or "managed." Therefore, the power is in the paradigm; that is why women who give birth unassisted at home generally have few complications. The only women in our society who will attempt this are women who are healthy and empowered. They are plugged into the paradigm.

It is precisely this paradigm that the medical birth community has so far been unable or unwilling to consider. In the same way that Semmelweis' contemporaries were unwilling to consider the radical notion that disease may not be a specific entity that could be distinctly correlated both clinically and pathologically, modern physicians are unwilling to consider the radical notion that childbirth is not a disease at all. Both of these ideologies persist/ed in spite of the overwhelming data disproving them. Both of these ideologies persist/ed as manifestations of a belief system that was inherited without being adequately exposed to the light of critical thinking and compelling scientific data.

But on a deeper level, the problems that medicine has encountered in attempting to be the sole managers of childbirth are an unavoidable expression of the intrinsic incompatibility of the two. The application of a Pathologization paradigm to a non-pathological body process is incongruent; it has always produced problems and inferior results and it always will. The answer for us today is the same answer as Semmelweis failed to recognize in 1847: The only way to truly address the massive problems medicine encounters in birth and health care is to honestly reexamine the limitations of the relationship itself.

The problem with The First Clinic in Vienna was not a lack of hand washing; the problem was the First Clinic of Vienna itself. The problem was the fundamental incompatibility of medicine and (normal) birth. On a certain level, by solving the wrong problem, Semmelweis merely perpetuated this dysfunctional relationship and framed the relentless problems associated with hospital birth in the context of a scientific answer waiting to be discovered, rather than a paradigm shift that was screaming to take place.

CHAPTER 7

The Midwife Problem: The Appropriation of Childbirth

Mothers tell your children,
Be quick you must be strong,
Life is full of wonder,
Love is never wrong,
Remember what they taught you,
How much of it was fear,
Refuse to hand it down,
The Legacy
Stops here.
-Melissa Etheridge

n late 19th and early 20th century United States, the scene was the same as Semmelweis' Germany and Hungary: midwives experiencing superior results, hospital births reeling with iatrogenic disease. The only difference is, in this case, the medical community was not only ignoring them, it was attacking them.

Even though the U.S. represented a less developed professional community, midwifery still managed childbirth with fewer complications and fewer deaths.[131] The simple explanation for this phenomenon is that midwives had superior training, superior experience, and furthermore were the more intrinsically appropriate care provider for the physiological process of birth than a surgeon, who is a specialist in pathology (disease and illness).

The fact that birth was safer before taking place in the hospitals, and that, even in the scientifically primordial era of 19th and early 20th century medicine, midwives were conducting safer, cleaner, and more expeditious births than the most educated and well financed hospitals is, for many, a difficult and painful reality to grasp.

For most of the scientific world, this was a painful but nevertheless inescapable reality. In 1902, the Midwife Protection Act was passed in Britain,[132] the beginning of a broad scale integration of midwifery care into the birth protocols of Europe, Scandinavia, and ultimately Asia and the rest of the developed world. Those countries would go on to develop birthing systems that would embarrass the U.S. in terms of safety and efficacy.

The U.S. took a radically different path. Midwifery was not codified and integrated; instead, it was co-opted and banished.

Today, childbirth in the U.S. is conducted differently than in any other industrialized nation. Most births in virtually every other developed country are managed by midwives, not doctors. Whereas Americans see midwives as backwards, hippie, counter-culture figures that are unscientific and risky, every other country sees them as simply the best birth attendants possible. The evidence is in their favor: As cited earlier, the U.S. ranks last or next to last in virtually every statistical measurement of safety and health in birth, from infant mortality to maternal mortality. In the case of the latter, the U.S. has the worst rates of any developed nation despite having the highest rates of medical care and intervention.

Marsden Wagner writes in *Born in the USA:*

"Twenty-eight countries have lower maternal mortality rates (women dying around the time of birth) than we do, and for more than 25 years the number of women dying around the time of birth in the United States has been increasing. Every year, at least one thousand women—that is, three jumbo jets full of our sisters, daughters, and mothers— die around the time of childbirth, and at least half of those deaths could have been prevented. Forty-one countries have lower infant mortality rates (babies dying before their first birthday)...It is important to note that in every country that has a lower maternal mortality rate than the United States—or a lower infant mortality rate—it is the midwives, not obstetricians, who manage normal pregnancies and births."[133]

How did we come to such a solitary, and so terribly unsuccessful, approach to childbirth?

How did we come to the place where the United States sees 95% to 99% of all births taking place in hospitals, managed by surgeons (obstetricians), while the rest of the civilized world sees 70% or more of births taking place out of the hospital, managed by midwives?

More importantly, how has this system been allowed to perpetuate when the data clearly does not support this practice?

The story of Ignaz Semmelweis should help you to comprehend this phenomenon. There is much to be praised and honored in medicine, but its social and cultural ascent was forged in, and continues to engender, a surrender of individual judgment. It is critical, despite the continuing faith that we are encouraged to hold in the science behind medical procedures, that we continue to exercise a healthy skepticism toward them. As we will see in Chapter 21, even today as few as one third of common medical practices have been proven by science to be effective and safe.

In order to understand how birth got into and has stayed in the hospitals, it is necessary to understand the unique and strange history behind medicalized childbirth in the United States. This story is important because it describes the true beginning of the intentional Pathologization of birth. Telling this story is invaluable in piecing together an understanding of how we can discuss reinventing our health care system in alignment with a more balanced view of humans and health.

The popular notion is that medicine, through superior methods and results, gained favor by producing improved methods; lives were saved, quacks were exposed, science won out, and medicine rose to the top.

The reality is far more complex. While American medical science did advance significantly in the 19th and 20th centuries, in the case of birth, the movement from the home to the hospital occurred not because of the results, but in spite of them.

Midwifery in Europe and the U.S. enjoyed a continuum of social standing and respect dating from the Middle Ages, and as late as 1900, 95% of all births, even in the U.S., were home births with midwives. But whereas in Europe, the success of midwifery care was recognized and supported by legislation such as the Midwife Protection Act, which established a framework for the licensing and education of midwives in Europe, in the U.S. a different opportunity was recognized.

Within the span of just a few decades, the place of birth for American women would go from 95% home births under the care of midwives to 95% hospital births under the care of surgeons.

It's natural for us in the U.S. to assume that the movement of birth into the hospital was a process driven by the scientific and technological superiority of modern medicine. It therefore can be difficult for many of us to learn that at the time of this transition, midwives were achieving superior results, with less trauma, intervention, and deaths in birth, than medical men were in hospitals.

In fact, the movement of birth into hospitals in the early 20th century cost the lives of thousands of American women. This was largely due to the continued prevalence of intrusive medical interventions and puerperal fever.

Historians Wertz and Wertz note:

"U.S. midwives caused no recorded epidemics of childbed fever among their patients... A distinguished medical historian of Virginia has calculated that the illiterate black midwives of that state spread less infection than did doctors until the end of the 19th century..."[134]

Even poorly trained lay midwives of the colonial period demonstrated higher levels of safety and success when it came to birth than most medical doctors. The records abound with evidence of the efficiency and safety of midwives as birth attendants:

- Mrs. Martha Moore Ballard, a midwife in Hallowell, Maine from 1778 to 1812, delivered 996 women with only four maternal deaths. She practiced for nine years before seeing her first maternal death.[135]
- Mrs. Thomas Whitmore, of Marlboro, Vermont, never lost a woman in the course of attending 2,000 births.[136]
- Midwife Hannah Porn, who was ultimately jailed for illegally continuing to practice midwifery after the medical coup was completed, maintained mortality rates HALF that of her medical colleagues during the eleven years and 642 births she attended.[137]

One of the reasons midwives were superior birth attendants was the fact that obstetrical training at the time was remedial at best.

Childbirth expert Ina May Gaskin writes:

"How little U.S. doctors themselves knew about labor and birth during the early twentieth century is evident by a 1912 study of obstetric education in 120 medical schools carried out by J. Whitridge Williams, an influential textbook author whose book, Williams Obstetrics, *is in its twenty-third edition at the time of this writing. This scathing report found an "appallingly slight experience, which many had before being appointed to professorships." Of his own institution, Johns Hopkins, Williams wrote, "I would unhesitatingly state that my own students are unfit on graduation to practice obstetrics in its*

broad sense, and are scarcely prepared to handle normal cases." Historian Judith Walzer Leavitt wrote, "Williams found that most medical students had the opportunity during their training to watch only one woman deliver, and one quarter of the medical schools admitted that their graduates were not competent to practice obstetrics."[138]

It is critical to fully apprehend the primitive nature of medicine in general, and obstetrical medicine, of this time. Bloodletting was still a common practice and appeared in obstetrical textbooks of the time. Cases exist of women being bled as many as 50 to 90 times throughout their pregnancy, and bloodletting was even used as a treatment for hemorrhage![139] Doctors insisted that women labor on their backs, a position which makes birthing far more difficult and complicated, and the use of interventions such as forceps was arbitrary and brutish. Of the forceps, William Hunter, an 18th century obstetrician commented, "Where they save one, they murder twenty."[140]

Many medical doctors of the time acknowledged the fact that the training and experience of midwives was superior to that of physicians. Williams' study cited above excoriated the entire medical profession, but saved its most scathing criticism for obstetrics, which made "the very worst showing,"[141] not helped by the almost total absence of actual clinical experience.[142] It was, in fact, this experience that physicians sought to co-opt from the midwives. Moving birth to the hospital represented a strategic appropriation of labor and delivery service privileges by a politically organized US obstetrical corps from a politically vulnerable and poorly organized community of midwives.

Faith Gibson, of the American College of Domiciliary Midwives, conducted a study of public health record data for this period of American history. She accessed archival records of professional journals from Stanford University Medical Library, which offer insight into the covert dialogue around the effort to replace the midwife. The following are some excerpts from her research[143]:

- The master plan to abolish midwives was not based on any categorical deficiency of midwives or a new medical "discovery" that made the principles and skills of traditional midwifery obsolete. Historically, in the U.S. and elsewhere, the practice of midwives was safer than the same kind of care as provided by physicians.
- Of the babies attended by midwives, 25.1 per 1000...died before the age of one month; of those attended by physicians, 38.2 per 1000...died before the

age of one month; and of those delivered in hospitals, 57.3 per 1000 died before the age of one month. These figures certainly <u>refute</u> the charge of high mortality among the infants whose mothers are attended by midwives, and instead *present the <u>unexpected problem</u> of explaining the fact that the maternal and infant mortality for the cases attended by midwives is lower than those attended by physicians and hospitals."* [1917-B, Levy, M.D.; p. 44 {emphasis added}

- The diagnostic ability of midwives is generally good and in the case of many, remarkable excellent. In this respect, the average midwife is fully the equal of the average physician." [Van Blarcom, M.D.; 1913]
- Clearly, the midwife seemed to be the safest birth attendant. [DeVitt, M.D.; 1975]

The American Journal of Clinical Nutrition described this period:

"Maternal mortality rates were very high in countries, states, regions, or areas where most deliveries were performed by physicians, especially in the hospital. Maternal mortality rates were also high when maximum surgical interference in normal or potentially normal labors was encouraged or advocated.[144]

The Journal of Surgery, Gynecology, and Obstetrics stated in 1922:

Our medical publications of the past century are rich in their contributions, but today, paradoxical as it may seem, the United States, of the more civilized countries, has the worst as well as the best in obstetrical practice. At least the investigation of Dr. Meigs of the Children's Bureau indicates that of sixteen civilized countries, the statistics of which have been studied, we stand fourteenth in deaths from childbirth.

Prior to the observations of Holmes and Semmelweis, the history of hospital maternities is to a great extent one of childbed fever...Today, we have ample proof from the records of many maternities that puerperal sepsis is a preventable complication. The continued large number of deaths from it is certainly a strong indication of general medical conditions..."[145]

The Kentucky Frontier Nursing Service, which provided midwifery-based care, is one organization that kept meticulous records during this period. Maternal mortality rates during deliveries between 1925 and 1937, compared with maternal mortality rates in other local and general populations of the United States in the same period, are below shown to be significantly lower than hospital births for women in that region:

Population	Maternal mortality rate (deaths/100000 births)
Women delivered by the KY Frontier Nursing Service	**60–70**
White women of Kentucky	440–530
White women delivered by physicians in hospitals in the city of Lexington, KY	800–900
United States	
Total	560–700
White	510–630
Nonwhite	900–1200

In 1931, the Committee on Prenatal and Maternal Care testified before the White House Conference on Child Health and Protection on the safety and effectiveness of midwifery and the dangers of delivering childbirth into the hands of surgeons:

"...that untrained midwives approach and trained midwives surpass the record of physicians in normal deliveries has been ascribed to several factors. Chief among these is the fact that the circumstances of modern practice induce many physicians to employ procedures which are calculated to hasten delivery, but which sometimes result in harm to mother and child. On her part, the midwife is not permitted to and does not employ such procedures. She waits patiently and lets nature take its course."[146] *(original emphasis)*

The second, unspoken but understood part of the Handy Hammer axiom is: Using a hammer for something other than nailing will usually cause more harm than good.

Nevertheless, the medical community organized a smear campaign against midwives, with the overt objective being to "eliminate" what was called "the Midwife Problem."

At the Sixth Annual Meeting of the American Association for Study and Prevention of the Infant Mortality in Philadelphia in November, 1915, Joseph Bolivar DeLee, the Father of Modern Obstetrics, presented his arguments for the abolishment of the midwife:

"I desire to state that I am fundamentally opposed to any movement designed to perpetuate the midwife. These are the grounds.

I.   *The midwife destroys obstetric ideals. She is a drag on our progress as a science and art.*
II. *The midwife is not absolutely necessary at the present time.*
III. *It is impossible to train the midwife sufficiently to make her a safe person to attend labor cases."*

DeLee presented no statistical evidence to support these premises, and in fact the data does not appear to have been on his side.

Of this era, Dr. Neal DeVitt, M.D. [1975] remarked that, "Most of the medical men had too much contempt for the midwife and too little respect for fact. The quality of the debate was poor. Evidence against the midwife was largely anecdotal or unsubstantiated opinion."[147]

In fact, the political and social attacks on the early American midwives were likely empowered by a deep cultural continuum with the infamous witch-hunts of the 14th to 17th century: a large number of the women who were burned at the stake by the thousands in Europe were, in fact, midwives. Indeed, it was in many cases the knowledge and practice of midwifery which implicated them in the first place. As midwives, they often possessed knowledge and expertise about the human body and natural remedies which were considered so esoteric and arcane that their possession—by a woman particularly—represented a direct and lethal threat to the governing force of medieval Europe, the Catholic Church.

"No one does more harm to the Church than midwives," wrote witch hunters Kramer and Sprenger.[148]

"The confusion of an earth-based, pagan religion called Wicca, or 'witchcraft,' with the practice of midwifery was simple enough...witchcraft was associated with magic, while the powers of midwives came from their special skills, including the use of herbs to heal and to end unwanted pregnancy,"[149] according to Suzanne Arms in *Immaculate Deception.*

The persecution and mass eradication of midwives in the Middle Ages and early modern period was not only a story of superstition, religion and mass hysteria, but also a story about power, and the instinct to protect power once it has been achieved. The most powerful social and political force in this era was the Catholic Church. The realms of both politics and medicine were governed by the Church. And the pogrom against witches and midwives resulted in a shift in power which enabled the emergence of the early European medical profession.

Barbara Ehrenreich writes more about it in *Witches, Midwives, and Nurses*[150]:

"The other side of the suppression of witches as healers was the creation of a new male medical profession, under the protection and patronage of the ruling classes. This new European medical profession played an important role in the witch-hunts, supporting the witches' persecution with "medical" reasoning:

"...Because the Medieval Church, with the support of kings, princes, and secular authorities, controlled medical education and practice, the Inquisition [witch-hunts] constitutes, among other things, an early instance of the "'professional' repudiating the skills and interfering with the rights of the 'nonprofessional' to minister to the poor." (Thomas Szasz, The Manufacture of Madness)

Gibson notes the inter-professional dialogue around the midwifery elimination campaign was similarly bereft of evidence and heavy on demonization and vague moral undertones:

"Any scheme for improvement in obstetric teaching and practice which does not contemplate the ultimate elimination of the midwife will not succeed. This is not alone because midwives can never be taught to practice obstetrics successfully, but most especially because of the moral effect upon obstetric standards. ['The Teaching of Obstetrics,' American Association of Obstetrics and Gynecologists.]"

This theme of establishing political power in the field of health care by means of force rather than reason is one that seems to have informed the appropriation of childbirth from the midwives of early America. The depiction of midwives as circumspect, suspicious, and untrustworthy in the 19th and 20th centuries, and the justification for their "eradication" is a part of a legacy of persecution that was already deeply ingrained in the psyche of the European mind. Both involved the manipulation of mass opinion. Both involved a group of men targeting a group of women. Both capitalized on a population (women) who had little political or social power to defend themselves. On a deeper level, the Witch Hunts and the Elimination of the Midwife all utilized their own version of Pathologization: the re-framing of normal into abnormal in this case, the Pathologization or demonization of a group of people who represented a perceived threat.

Historian Renate Blumenfeld-Kosinski wrote, "The professionalization of medicine and the Witch Hunts worked together to ensure a male control over women in medicine."[151]

Because the appropriation of childbirth from the midwives was certainly not driven by compelling evidence.

Gibson's data shows that:

*"During this long period of inadequately trained doctors (1910 to the early 1930s) maternal mortality in the US rose from a baseline in 1900 of **665:100,000**, to a high of **1,200 death per 100,000 in 1925**. Out of two million live births in 1925, there were 25,000 maternal deaths reported (**one out of 80**)."*

How do we explain the motivations of this campaign, if it cannot be supported by scientific data?

"... the basis of the campaign to eliminate the 'un-American midwife' was the self-interest of obstetricians. The primary issue of self-interest was the desire of the obstetricians to expand the influence and increase the status of their specialty. During this period obstetricians worried constantly about the status of their profession." [DeVitt, M.D., 1975]

"Legalizing the midwife will...work a definite hardship to those physicians who have become well-trained in obstetrics, for it will have a definite tendency to decrease their sphere of influence." [Huntington, M.D., 1913]

It would be unfair, though, to characterize the midwife smear campaign as purely self-interest. The period during which the major anti-midwife movement occurred was also a time, fueled by the Flexner Report in 1908, that the medical establishment was seeking to reform its profession by increasing its standards for education and training. Obstetrics was a field conspicuously lacking.

The obstetrician occupied an unenviable status even among physicians.

While modern-day observers would note that modern obstetrics enjoys great professional status, it must be remembered that "Man-Midwifery," as it was called throughout out the 17th, 18th, and 19th centuries, was considered the poor step-sister of "modern-medicine," cast aside as a dubious form of "woman's work" not worthy of the attention of formally-educated "medical men."

Many physicians shunned obstetrics as a specialty, and obstetric care was provided by poorly trained or untrained medical practitioners.[152]

During the height of the midwife elimination campaign, physicians exploited the vulnerable status of midwife as both woman and non-physician. They thus required neither science nor facts in order to conduct this eradication. It was merely a question of "enhancing" the framework of birth to be washed of any remaining semblance of normality, so that it naturally would fall under the aegis of heroic medicine.

Physicians' access to the technologies that lent social gravitas to their cultural campaign was not their only advantage. The illiteracy rates among women in the early 20th century and lack of access to texts was also a factor, along with a poorly developed communication network. Starr adds:

"Doctors' access to and ultimate control of knowledge concerning birth are, in the final analysis, the most potent factors in explaining why birth became a medical event. In the nineteenth century...doctors developed an extensive and effective communications network—a network from which women were largely excluded... As alternative practitioners were eliminated and alternative models of birth management discredited... and as birth moved out of the home and into the hospital, American women came to depend on medicine as the only source of knowledge about a central female experience."[153]

The public relations scheme included two components: the smear campaign against the midwives and a characterization of hospitals as clean and safe. This is of course ironic because at the time, the hospital was anything but clean OR safe. Childbed fever was caused by a lack of cleanliness and its incidence was far higher in hospitals than at home.

That truth did not stop the campaign's effectiveness, however, as the growing cultural authority of the medical profession was already leading to what Starr called "the retreat of private judgment." The public was, more and more, willing to "trust their doctors".

The immediate effect of the movement of birth into the hospital was a dramatic increase in morbidity and mortality.

The CDC reports:

Maternal mortality rates were highest in this century during 1900-1930. **Poor obstetric education and delivery practices were mainly responsible for the high numbers of maternal deaths, most of which were preventable** *[my emphasis]...Inappropriate and excessive surgical and obstetric interventions (e.g., induction of labor, use of forceps, episiotomy, and cesarean deliveries) were common and increased during the 1920s. Deliveries, including some surgical interventions, were performed without following the principles of asepsis. As a result, 40% of maternal deaths were caused by sepsis...*[154]

The widespread utilization of surgical and technological interventions in labor and delivery were always a hallmark of obstetrical practice, especially since early obstetricians were usually called in only when the situation had become so dire that the fetus had to be killed and extracted in order to save the life of the mother. But as obstetricians vied for a larger share of normal births, the continued use of these interventions (and the presence of the surgeons who wielded them) needed justification. That justification would be articulated in the form of an argument for the "pathologic dignity" of pregnancy and birth: their Pathologization.

And the spokesperson for the Pathologization of Birth was a man by the name of Joseph Bolivar DeLee.

CHAPTER 8

The Pathologization of Childbirth: The Delee Protocols

Joseph DeLee is known as "the father of modern obstetrics." His influence on medicine and maternity was so significant he was featured on the cover of Time magazine in 1936.

His radical plan for universal surgical childbirth involved drugging the mother, cutting open her birth canal, and forcefully extracting the fetus with steel forceps. While DeLee remains today a pariah of the natural childbirth community, his notions can be seen as nothing more than the natural consequence of the questionable union of surgical specialists and the normal process of birth.

Joseph DeLee was born in 1869, one of 10 children in a Jewish immigrant family living in Cold Springs, New York. His father did not want him to become a surgeon, but rather a rabbi, but his mother supported his medical aspirations.

DeLee's immediate goal upon completing his training was to use medical science to address the persistently high maternal mortality rates that continued to plague American hospitals. Despite the fact that improved hygiene and public health had made significant advances in the spread of infectious diseases in the general population and in rural and urban areas, maternal mortality in US hospitals remained unimproved from the 1800s until as late as the mid 1940s. Much of this mortality was caused by postpartum infection, which many scientists of DeLee's era reasoned should have declined concomitantly with the decline of infections elsewhere, as knowledge of infectious disease and germs crystallized. However, this was not the case, and women continued to perish in hospital maternity wards at alarming rates.

DeLee's radical views on obstetrical interventions were clearly influenced by his experiences as a very young doctor working at a Chicago baby farm. The illegitimate children unlucky enough to be born there suffered a staggeringly high rate of mortality, often from cerebral hemorrhage as a result of difficult deliveries. DeLee, whose belief, like many of his peers, in the absolute power of medicine to solve all of the world's problems was virtually complete and unquestioning, sought to apply the limitless potential of medical knowledge to the problem of maternal mortality.

DeLee's experience in birth was so dramatic that he came to adopt a peculiar—and highly controversial—view of pregnancy and childbirth. In 1920, DeLee wrote an article for the first edition of the new American Journal of Obstetrics and Gynecology entitled, *The Prophylactic Forceps Operation*. In it he states,

"So frequent are these bad effects that I have often wondered whether Nature did not deliberately intend women should be used up in the process of reproduction, in a manner analogous to that of salmon, which dies after spawning?"

It was in this now famous treatise that DeLee proposes that all births be managed with sedatives, surgery, and instrumentation. DeLee goes on to present his unusual perspective on the process of birth; namely, as a pathology:

"Perhaps laceration, prolapse and all the evils [to which women in labor are subjected] are, in fact, natural to labor and therefore normal, in the same way as the death of the mother salmon and the death of the male bee in copulation are natural and normal. If you adopt this view, I have no ground to stand on, but if you believe that a woman after delivery should be as healthy, as well, as anatomically perfect as she was before, and that the child should be undamaged, then you will have to agree with me that labor is pathogenic, because experience has proved such ideal results exceedingly rare."

This is an astonishingly unscientific system of thinking for establishing medical protocols. He states that, "Labor is pathogenic because experience has proved ideal results rare." DeLee aggressively pursues the adoption of massive universal changes in obstetrical protocol purely based on his own limited professional experience. No studies were cited, no scientific evidence referenced. Furthermore, and more importantly, DeLee had virtually no experience with how birth looks when it takes place naturally, is managed with a different (non-medical) set of protocols. He did, however, have knowledge of two important facts: First, that home birth with midwives represented

60% of the births in the U.S. at his time; and second, that these births had superior outcomes than hospital births.

At the time, only 10 percent of women in the Chicago area gave birth in hospitals. It was generally regarded as a last resort for unwed mothers and the poor,[155] hardly a representative sample. Not only were the cases to which DeLee was exposed generally of uncommonly poor health and state of mind, but the mere fact that they were in a hospital environment certainly impacted the birth outcomes. Mortality rates in hospital births were, after all, as we have seen, higher than home births with midwives. Hospital environments and procedures can also negatively impact birth outcomes, as we will also see later. Understanding these factors is critical if we are to understand fully why DeLee's measures were not only inadequately informed, but ultimately, failures.

Professionally, obstetrics at this time occupied a rather innocuous, often belittled place in the pantheon of medical hierarchy. They were the product of a legacy of physicians whose craft had been perpetually undervalued by both the public and even their own peers.

They confronted, too, the fundamental incongruity of their relationship with normal childbirth. Physicians had no training for "normal." Theirs was a profession of life-saving, of heroic intervention upon the ailing and sickly, with the promise of recovery.

But pregnant women aren't "ailing." They are not sick at all. The existence of every person on the planet is a testament to the normalcy of childbirth. Such is the dilemma facing the obstetrician of 1920. What is a surgeon doing managing a person who is not sick?

DeLee's answer is simply to re-define "sick."

Specifically, he argues for childbirth, one of the most self-evidently fundamental human biological processes imaginable, to now be called a disease.

It is for DeLee's argument for the "pathologic dignity" of childbirth that he is perhaps most well-known.

"Labor has been called, and still is believed by many, to be a normal function. [Y]et it is a decidedly pathologic process...if a woman falls on a pitchfork, and drives the handle through her perineum, we call that pathologic-abnormal, but if a large baby is driven through the pelvic floor, we say that is natural, and therefore normal. If a baby were to have its head caught in a door very lightly, but enough to cause cerebral hemorrhage, we would say that it is decidedly pathologic, but when a baby's head is crushed against a tight pelvic floor, and a hemorrhage in the brain kills it, we call this normal."

DeLee's proposal here is monumental. Imagine a gastroenterologist publishing a paper arguing for the digestion of food to now be classified as a pathology which requires the constant and intensive intervention of a gastroenterologist and you will have an idea as to both the boldness and the blatant conflict of interest inherent in DeLee's notorious comments.

This audacious and perhaps self-serving re-framing also planted the seeds of the eventual story that our current society holds around medicine and birth, which is that birth was dangerous until doctors saved it. This story is a natural by-product of the Pathologization of birth. If women who are pregnant are "sick," then naturally they should, like any sick person, rely on a physician's help. Physicians, from 1920 to the present, have consequently argued for greater and greater medical intervention in birth, greater and greater medical technology, and greater and greater authority and exclusive rights to pre- and post-natal care. The problem is, it didn't work, because pregnancy does not become an illness simply because a man calls it an illness. But that doesn't mean people didn't listen.

The growing social status of the physician, and the fact that pregnancy and child-birth represented a clinical relationship between a physician, a person of significant social standing and authority, and a woman, a person who had the legal rights of a child only a few years previously, meant that the capacity of the physician to control the relationship was vast. Thus, the continuation of the trend from home to hospital birth was driven by powerful social and political factors, some self-serving and some earnestly philanthropic in intent. However, the one factor that did not support the movement of birth into the hospital was science. Hospital births were more danger-ous in 1920, and they did not get safer any time soon. But science did not stop Joseph DeLee or the emerging cartel of the obstetrical field.

There were three parts to DeLee's formula for medical birth management:

1. Universal sedation of women.
2. Universal episiotomy.
3. Universal forceps extraction of fetus.

The radical notion of DeLee's proposals was not intervention in birth, of course, but intervention without indications. The only way to justify this measure was to simply redefine childbirth itself. For birth as a normal physiological event to be subjected to the universal treatment of surgeons, doctors who are trained in medical emergencies, represents an inescapable incongruence. But birth re-defined as a disease naturally places it, with mother and child both intrinsically endangered, in the realm of the heroic physician, the obstetrician.

What is most astounding about Joseph DeLee's recommendations is that, despite initial criticism, they were ultimately adopted wholeheartedly by the medical community. Even Williams' own textbook reflected the subtle transformation. While the fourteenth edition divides normal from abnormal conditions of pregnancy and delivery, the fifteenth, sixteenth, and seventeenth editions gradually erase the lines between the normal and abnormal. Unfortunately, the implementation of the DeLee measures was not supported by the scientific results.

A sounder scientific approach to the question of how to manage birth would be to create a representative picture of what birth looked like, how it proceeded, and the intrinsic problems or dangers that might exist, before seeking to solve those problems or propose new protocols. This picture would be represented not only by hospital births, but by home births with lay midwives, professional midwives, and general practitioners. This system of gathering information is based on a fundamental scientific principle, that if you change the conditions of the experiment, you can change the results.

We now know with certainty that "birth," for any woman, is not some embedded recording that will simply "play out" once the start button is pushed. The physiology of birth is governed by the tenuous and fickle flow of body chemicals, many of which in turn are influenced by a mass of factors, from the woman's state of mind, to the ambient temperature, to her sense of safety and privacy, to even the level of light in the room. Every one of her senses, in fact, is a sophisticated trigger that can either facilitate or arrest the flow of birth-dependent hormones. To discount the location and conditions of the birth process from a characterization of birth itself would be like taking the blood pressures of the entire floor of traders on Wall Street one minute before closing bell and using that data as representative of American blood pressure.

DeLee's fatal error is that he manufactured his picture of birth from the *minority* data, rather than the *majority*. Dismissing the work and results of a massive population of female caregivers was hardly a radical act in 1920, when women had only recently earned the right to vote. Even Semmelweis had made that mistake. And DeLee's personal experiences of birth were probably so vivid and dramatic that one can imagine them instilling in him a powerful motivation for reform. In his article, "The Prophylactic Forceps Operation," he cites a four percent death rate for infants, even with the protections of modern obstetrics.[156] This rate is clearly a poor representation of birth from a biological standard, and more likely an aberration of enculturated forces acting upon that process, not the least of which, clearly, was medicine itself.

And as Semmelweis did seventy years earlier, DeLee dismissed the most obvious answer before him: to utilize the system, which was producing the best results, and improve, replicate, and standardize it. This is indeed what the rest of the civilized world did. But even at the dawn of women's suffrage, this gesture of acknowledgement to a cultural and sexual minority and professional competitor was beyond the capacity of any typical physician of his era.

DeLee certainly publicly admitted that the state of obstetrics in the U.S. was dismal, and that women and children suffered for it. He also pointed to the midwives as a profession, which was unregulated and delivered inconsistent results, a charge not entirely without merit. However, like most of his contemporaries, DeLee believed that to improve the standards of midwife care was wholly impractical; besides, it would be an initiative that would rob his own profession of a vast and perpetually renewing source of revenue. His faith in the growing power and knowledge of medicine was vast, and he placed the future of obstetrical care in his profession, to the rigorous exclusion of midwifery.

It seems hard to believe that DeLee would have had no access to the fact that improvement, standardization, and licensing of midwives had already been accomplished with excellent results in Europe. The Midwife Protection Act in Britain helped to successfully establish the very conditions DeLee and his contemporaries refused to consider: safe home and hospital births managed by trained midwives delivering superior results at reduced cost and with reduced complications.

However, his proposals—the routine and universal use of scopolamine, ether, episiotomy, and forceps—were a radical suggestion even for the highly medicalized hospital birth environment. They were soundly rejected by DeLee's colleague, J. Whitridge Williams, author of the authoritative manual on the subject, *Williams' Obstetrics*. He said, "If I have understood Dr. DeLee correctly, it seems to me that he interferes 19 times too often out of 20."[157]

In his last edition of *Obstetrics*, Williams stated, regarding the DeLee protocols, "I am confident that the results would be disastrous were (his) suggestions generally adopted." Ultimately, astonishingly, DeLee's suggestions would indeed be adopted. The 1936 edition of *Obstetrics* had the line dropped, and by 1950 the recommendations were accepted without reservation.

A 1933 report on maternal mortality published by the Commonwealth Fund in New York stated:

"The great increase in the hospitalization of the normal parturient has failed to bring the hoped-for reduction in puerperal morbidity and mortality, and this in spite of great advances in our knowledge of the processes involved and the proper way of treating them. It would seem that the present attitude toward home confinement requires re-examination..."

Later in the study, which compared, perhaps for the first time, the outcomes of midwife-attended births and physician-attended births in an unbiased manner, the authors bluntly concluded:

"To the Committee it seems fair to say that contrary to the generally accepted opinion, the midwife is an acceptable attendant for properly selected cases of labor and delivery... we have seen that her results are as good as those obtained by the physician under what are justly regarded as comparable circumstances and for comparable cases."[158]

The DeLee protocols institutionalized surgical intervention in all, even perfectly healthy and normal births. (This category, essentially, was made extinct by DeLee: all births were pathological. Even today, we do not use the term "safe" or "normal" but only speak of birth in terms of relative risk: "high risk" and "low risk.") And while these interventions may have been clinically defensible in rare cases, used universally, they institutionalized trauma and complications for women and their babies.

The Forceps

The first of the DeLee protocols I'd like to discuss are the forceps (even though, in the chronology of birth, they are used last). Forceps are a tool composed of two metal blades, jointed midway, similar to salad tongs. The instrument is inserted into the birth canal, the blades positioned on either side of the infant's skull. Pressure exerted on the opposite end, the "handles," thus created a strong gripping force. The "user" then squeezes the forceps, pulls, and twists the cranium of the baby.

This tool was first widely used in 1588. The inventor, Peter Chamberlin, maintained a fanatically jealous secrecy over the design of the instrument. Only members of his family were allowed access to the use of the forceps, a practice which continued successfully until the death of the last living descendant, Dr. Hughes Chamberlin, in 1728. During that time, when the forceps were used by one of the Chamberlins (assuming the patient's family could afford the exorbitant fee), the entire procedure was accomplished in secret: the forceps kept in a locked box, opened under the sheet which covered the woman's genitalia, assembled blindly, used, and replaced, all invisibly.[159]

The release of the esoteric "iron fingers" into the greater birthing community saw a marked increase in its use. The previously mentioned factors—rickets, corsets, and nutritional and overall health and wellness deficiencies—meant that protracted labor was abnormally high. In some of these cases, the forceps were the most useful tool available, and indeed seemed to help. Of course, their use was still based on the presence of clinical factors indicating their need, namely, protracted labor.

"Prophylactic obstetrics" meant a change in the clinical criteria for the use of forceps, or, more accurately, the *removal* of clinical criteria for their use. Under the DeLee protocol, forceps would be utilized in the absence of any clinical indicators of their need. It was this aspect of DeLee's proposal that concerned some of his peers as much as any other. Medicine, until now, had operated on the premise that intervention was appropriate based on clinical indicators. DeLee argued that waiting for those indicators wasted valuable time, and it was better to apply the heroic measures universally and preemptively (prophylactically). But many of his contemporaries saw danger in such thinking. The evidence would ultimately vindicate their concerns.

Use of forceps does not go without risks. There are three vectors of force applied in forceps: the force applied to the baby's skull, the twisting force, and the pulling force. Each of these force applications, as well as each *combination* of force applications, engenders its own series of risks to the mother and baby.

Risks of forceps to the baby include: facial nerve damage, skull fracture, intracranial hemorrhage, facial paralysis, and bruising leading to jaundice after the birth. There is also a possibility of pulling the neck vertebrae out of alignment. These risks have much to do with the placement of the blades and the amount of traction the doctor uses.

Force application in forceps use has been measured at up to 110 pounds.[160] Take a moment to picture in your mind a newborn baby held upside down with a 100-pound weight hanging from his head. Now add rotation and lateral flexion of the neck to the picture and you may be able to imagine the potential for severe cervical trauma that forcible extraction can have for the fetus.

Risks to the mother include: lacerations of the pelvic floor and birth canal, urinary tract infection, and bladder or rectum injury with accompanying urinary or fecal incontinence. The most severe risks of forceps deliveries to babies include facial nerve damage[161] and spinal cord injury.[162] With facial nerve damage, permanent facial asymmetry may occur, especially evident when the child laughs or cries. Spinal cord damage is permanent and irreversible. Judicious utilization of forceps can undeniably facilitate difficult deliveries. There were, however, problems with the adoption of universal utilization of forceps:

1. It was adopted without any real data examining the potential risks of using forceps on patients who are not presenting with any indications of their need. In other words, no risk/benefit assessment was attempted.
2. It established, perpetuated, and enabled a larger paradigm of birth as intrinsically a crisis. The forceps were always an emergency intervention tool. The scientifically unsubstantiated universalization of their use implicitly reframed the deeper social sense of birth, and to a great degree pregnancy as a pathology.

The use of forceps became indelibly linked to the broader strategy of powerful drugs and episiotomy. The drugs provided a relief from the pain of childbirth but rendered the patient wholly incapable of participating in their own labor; the need for forceps thus became something of a self-fulfilling prophesy. Popular wisdom of the time considered the episiotomy, too, a necessary by-product of the tortuous nature of hospital birth, despite the glaring absence of any data to support this premise.

Episiotomy

The second element of DeLee's protocol was the routine episiotomy. In this procedure, the surgeon makes an incision in the perineum from the posterior aspect of the vagina towards the anus, or at an angle postero-laterally.

There are reports of the procedure being performed in England in the mid-1700s, but the first published account of episiotomy in a medical journal was in 1810. Use of the procedure was still inconsistent until after 1920.

The premise of the episiotomy is, on the surface, plausible: The surgeon widens the opening through which the fetus must pass in order to facilitate delivery. There are several realities, however, which have made the episiotomy a highly controversial and rapidly evaporating procedure.

First, there has never been any evidence to show that episiotomy facilitates delivery.

"A retrospective review was performed of the medical literature on outcomes for routine episiotomy between 1950 and 2004. Although long term outcomes could not be determined, the study showed not only no benefit from the episiotomy, but negative effects. Pain with intercourse was more common, and fecal and urinary incontinence were not prevented.
— JAMA 293(17): 2141–48, May 2005

"A presumed benefit of episiotomy is to protect the baby from the adverse consequences of an extended second stage of labour, including lack of oxygen and trauma to the head, which has been said to lead to cerebral palsy and mental retardation....

"In summary, 'There is no evidence to suggest that, when the second stage of labour is progressing and the condition of both mother and fetus is satisfactory, the imposition of any arbitrary upper limit on its duration is justified. Such limits should be discarded.' (Sleep, J. et al., 'Care during the second stage of labor,' in "Effective Care in Pregnancy and Childbirth.") Studies of [cerebral palsy and mental retardation] suggest that they originate for the most part before labour and birth. Neither of the two clinical trials which looked at this issue found any evidence that episiotomy reduces trauma to the fetal head. No surgical procedure, even one that seems rather trivial to the people who perform it, should be widely used without convincing evidence of benefit. As yet, no published study adequately proves the claimed benefits of episiotomy."
-Marsden Wagner M.D., *Pursuing the Birth Machine*, 1994

It is believed by many medical historians that the procedure simply evolved as a logical measure to take during protracted labor. DeLee's inclusion of episiotomy in his notorious protocol includes the argument that the mother's vagina could be surgically restored to what he called "virginal conditions."[163]

Modern science has, of course, dispelled the notion that vaginal birth must negatively impact the enjoyment of intercourse for either partner, and in fact accounts abound of the nightmare that overzealous post-operative suturing made of sexual intercourse for countless women.

JAMA reports:
"Evidence does not support maternal benefits traditionally ascribed to routine episiotomy. In fact, outcomes with episiotomy can be considered worse since some proportion of women who would have had lesser injury instead had a surgical incision. They also note pain with intercourse was more common among women with episiotomy."[164]

The effort to "restore virginal conditions" is an unusual one. It implies, of course, that the birth process is permanently damaging to the woman's sexual value, and that this value is somehow tied in with the concept of virginity. This story, of birth being intrinsically pathological, of the high cultural value associated with virginity, of birth being fundamentally evil in a sense because it represents the intractable end of virginity, has its roots deep in the psyche of Western man. The assumption, by men, of the role of arbiters and restorers of a woman's intrinsic sexual value, speaks of the cultural power male doctors enjoyed at this time. It is what Robbie Pfeufer Kahn cites as "the appropriation by men of women's sexual and reproductive capacity."

"The technological veil of medicine obscures how obstetric practice is a cultural, not just a medical, phenomenon...Accepting a definition of patriarchy as a social institution, the study of obstetric practice becomes a study of one of the most embodied forms of patriarchal control...Where once myth legitimated patriarchy, now science does."
  -Robbie Pfeufer Kahn, *Bearing Meaning*

"A basic belief of seventeenth-century Calvinism, a Protestant sect that heavily influenced Northern Europe for many years, and Puritanism, another Protestant sect of the same period that heavily influenced both Britain and its North American colonies, was that the female body was unclean and corrupt. The hallmark of Puritanism was its rigorous moral code, which emphasized strictness, austerity, and purity, and led directly to the suppression of all that was physical, including sex. Since it was never possible to give birth without being both physical and sexual, women were seen as essentially unclean...
  ...The degraded view of the female body continued into Victorian times and continues in our culture—and our medical practices—today. It affects all women, whether or not they consider themselves to be religious."
  -Suzanne Arms, *Immaculate Deception*

The story of the Virgin Mary and the myth of the Virgin Birth is a deeply evocative archetype of this enduring subconscious ethic. It solves the puzzle of how to establish the sanctity of Jesus' birth without invoking what Western religion had decreed to be fundamentally "unclean": sexuality and birth. The solution was to simply omit sexuality from the equation. Hence, the Immaculate Conception. Mary doesn't need to be restored to virginal conditions: She is the perpetual virgin. The image, perhaps out of place in today's modern world of science and technology, nevertheless speaks to how deep these ethics remain to modern man. At the same time, they are also vestiges of a worldview that was based on the oppression and abuse of women and the delegation of womankind to the status of a mere article of possession. The Pathologization of birth was a natural extension of a long lineage of Pathologizing women themselves that predates modern medicine itself. The idea of being *Born Broken* is nothing new to women throughout history: That genealogy can be traced all the way back to the Garden of Eden. In interpretations that emerged in modern re-translations of the Bible, Eve is implicated in the initiation of the corruption of all mankind and the establishment of Original Sin—the prototypical application of the paradigm *Born Broken*.

Ether and Scopolamine

The third of the DeLee protocols was universal sedation of women in labor. In his fight to universalize comprehensive aggressive surgical intervention in normal childbirth, DeLee would find a surprising and ultimately ironic ally: women.

The year is 1847. A Scottish physician by the name of Sir James Young Simpson has made a discovery that will change the face of medicine forever. While experimenting with friends, Simpson discovers the anesthetic properties of chloroform. Interestingly, Simpson was a staunch advocate of the presence of midwives in hospital births.

The advent of relatively safe and effective anesthesia transformed the field of medicine completely. Surgery had been largely limited to the extremities and superficial aspects of the body since the pain of more invasive procedures would so commonly cause shock or death. In the field of obstetrics, chloroform, and, later, morphine and scopolamine, would bring with them an opportunity for women to escape the significant physical pain and trauma of childbirth brought on by the conditions of 19th century pregnancy and labor practices.

After Queen Victoria famously gave birth to Prince Leopold with the aid of chloroform in 1853, its use as a surgical and obstetrical anesthetic quickly became widespread. Some opposition to this development existed at the time, based on an interpretation of the biblical verse "In sorrow thou shalt bring forth children." (Genesis 3:16)[165] The possibility of effective pain relief for labor was an irresistible concept for 19th century women.

For it indeed was women themselves who argued for, even demanded, access to painkilling drugs in childbirth.[166] When the drug cocktail of scopolamine, ether or chloroform, and morphine was developed to induce the now notorious "twilight sleep," it had mixed support among doctors, but strong support among women, who by now had lost all connection to the natural, safe, normal birth of their ancestors. All they knew was the pain, fear, and torture they were taught to expect (and, by some, to deserve) from childbirth, and Twilight Sleep, a state of amnesiatic unconsciousness in which the mother awoke from labor to find her baby being handed to her and no memory whatsoever of the experience, must have seemed like a godsend. The drugs were part of the DeLee protocol and initially supported by the public at large.

The Suffragists advocated twilight sleep as a basic woman's right. They formed groups, such as the National Twilight Sleep Association, to fight for access to scopolamine for labor pain relief.[167] One female homeopathic doctor, frustrated and angered by her own traumatic birth experiences, opened her own "Twilight Sleep Maternity Hospital in Boston, to offer the drug to mothers who were denied it by traditional hospitals."[168]

Indeed, there was significant opposition to the utilization of scopolamine in the medical realm.

But DeLee's camp, with the aid of the popular demand for what women perceived, or had been told, was safe and effective pain relief, ultimately won out.

The women who were advocating for twilight sleep had little knowledge of its actual effects. But after a series of letters to the editor were published in 1958 in *Ladies Home Journal* detailing the brutality witnessed in maternity wards while women were under twilight sleep, women began to fear what would be done to their bodies more than they feared the pain.

The heading of the *Journal* piece was "Cruelty in the Maternity Ward," and it provided a more detailed account of twilight sleep. Women who became delusional under the influence of the drug and had to be restrained with leather straps. Babies so sedated by the drugs that they had to be held upside down and slapped to revive them (so that's where that comes from!). Women being drugged without their consent and treated harshly, the skin being worn from their wrists and ankles from the wild thrashing about in labor.

The 1970 edition of a Nicholas Eastman book on childbirth described the drug cocktail's effect as such:

"A woman under twilight sleep may shriek, make grimaces and show other evidence of pain, but upon awakening from the drug will remember nothing about her labor and will vow that she experienced no pain whatsoever.

Thus it was the amnesiatic effects of the drugs that helped to perpetuate its use: women, having no memory of their own horrific experience, often expressed satisfaction with the process."[169]

Even Eastman neglected to point out that the drugs actually, according to Suzanne Arms in *Immaculate Deception*:

...induced a kind of wild psychosis in many women, who fought nurses, scratched themselves, or tried to throw themselves out of the bed. For this reason, the side rails of hospital beds were kept up, heavy leather pads were put inside to protect women from bruising themselves on the metal rails, and women were physically tied down. Many women were shocked to find themselves covered with bruises when they awoke after the birth, with no memory of the cause. Others found themselves completely hoarse, having no recall that they had lost their voice from screaming. Many harbored doubts that the baby they were shown was really theirs. This is the way many of our mothers, grandmothers, and great-grandmothers gave birth.[170]

The public outrage that these stories incited breathed life into what we now know as the natural childbirth movement. In 1944, Dr. Grantly Dick-Read's *Childbirth Without Fear* (which was actually written in 1933) was finally published in the U.S., and served as a siren call to a new manifestation of women's rights in birth.

But from 1914 to 1958, twilight sleep was a central factor in the story of childbirth in the U.S. Even the barbiturates, Seconal or Nebutal, which replaced scopolamine, are sleep-inducers which, according to Eastman, resulted in the woman "knowing nothing about her labor and awakening several hours after the baby had been born."

Understanding the forces driving the utilization of such dangerous and traumatizing drugs as scopolamine requires a deeper understanding of the experience of childbirth from the woman's perspective.

For most women of the early twentieth century, for their mothers, grandmothers, great-grandmothers, and so on for literally centuries, childbirth was a legacy of pain, torment, and peril. As we saw in Chapter 4, childbirth was not always this way. Birth was, for millennia, a short and easy affair, with no danger and threat to mother or child. That changed with certain developments in human culture and customs, and those changes compounded until the lore of pain and peril exceeded the reach of the legacy of normal, natural birth. Women, for the first time, had no access to the birth their own bodies had evolved to perform. All they knew was the pain and fear their mothers, sisters, and aunts experienced, and even dangerous and untested drugs like scopolamine were welcomed escapes from the legacy they faced.

Delee: Consequences, Inertia, and Scientism

The early and middle 20th century turned out to be a critical intersection in the Pathologization of Birth. As public health measures improved living conditions for birthing women, the ascension of the obstetrical profession and the promise of safer, easier births created a perfect storm which swept the medicalization of childbirth in America into full prominence, even as the continuum of normal, natural birth remained an invisible and mostly unrealized standard for women and babies.

The American natural childbirth movement, which may be said to have started in the 1930s with *Childbirth without Fear*, was slowed by the perceived relationship between improved childbirth outcomes and medicalized birth in the 1940s and 1950s. In 1900, 95% of births in the U.S. occurred at home. By 1955, 95% of all births occurred in hospitals.[171] And although the more grisly elements of Twilight Sleep had been eliminated, the Pathologization of Birth remained a constant. And Pathologization always has consequences.

Hospitalization of pregnant women in the 19th and 20th centuries led to an epidemic of monumental proportions. Medicalization of pregnant women in the 20th century engendered the establishment of a culture of institutionalized intervention, which systematically impeded the normal, healthy expression of the biological blueprint for birth. While the technologies have changed, the obstruction of normal labor and delivery continues, perhaps more so than ever.

DeLee's protocols did not, as he perhaps envisioned, save women's lives, but in fact, perpetuated high maternal mortality rates. He did, however, accomplish one of his goals: that of elevating the status of the obstetrician and the establishment of a virtual monopoly on childbirth for physicians.

However, characterizations of DeLee—by many detractors, particularly in the field of natural childbirth and women's rights—as a misogynistic villain often fall short of a well rounded perspective on the man. DeLee's attitudes about women were typical of the 1920s American male, and his bias against women's capabilities in childbirth was shared by many of his colleagues. One wrote in 1930 that "the tissues of the modern women do not well withstand the tension and stretching incident to the average normal labor,"[172] and DeLee himself called women "nervous, inefficient products of modern civilization."[173] DeLee was a fervent advocate for the safety and health of women and children. He truly seemed to believe that his proposals were in the best interest of women in general. Furthermore, the ultimate adoption of his protocols was aided by women's groups themselves, as we will see. Two years before he died, DeLee seemed to sense the Frankenstein's monster he had unleashed and warned the audience at a Mother's Day address to avoid doctors who attempted to rush the birth process. "Mother Nature's methods of bringing babies are still the best," he stressed belatedly.[174]

The problem with his position was that it was simply not scientific (although in his defense very little in medicine was at that time—the term "evidence-based medicine" would not even appear in medical literature until 1991). It was clearly based on his limited professional experience and biases. It failed to objectively assess the impact and potential of the midwives, an error that Europe, Scandinavia, and, ultimately, most of the rest of the industrialized world fortunately avoided. It also failed to objectively assess and apply the scientific data that did come in on how effective these protocols were once applied.

And while maternal mortality did indeed fall eventually in the U.S., though not until after 1950, it is aptly noted by many historians that the dramatic changes in hygiene, nutrition, and sanitation that occurred in the mid to late 20th century were largely responsible for these changes.

"...The pleasant story of scientific progress has been replaced by a darker tale of medical competitiveness and misplaced confidence in an imperfect science. Medical science did not, on the whole, increase women's chances of surviving childbirth until well into the twentieth century, the new histories argue, and may actually have increased the dangers."

–Laurel Thatcher Ulrich (James Duncan Phillips Professor of Early American history at Harvard University), from Women and Health in America: Historical Readings, edited by Judith Waltzer Leavitt

Richard and Dorothy Wertz note:

"The White House conference on child health and protection issued its report in 1933 entitled fetal, newborn, and maternal mortality and morbidity. It featured the fact that maternal mortality had not declined between 1915 and 1930 despite the increase in hospital delivery, the introduction of prenatal care, and more use of aseptic techniques. The number of infant deaths from birth injuries had actually increased by 40% to 50% from 1915 to 1929."[175]

The question you may be asking again here is how, if the results do not support them, do measures like these get perpetuated? Why aren't they discarded and replaced with more effective measures? Isn't that the way that scientific progress works?

"Reason is no abstract force pushing inexorably toward greater freedom at the end of history. Its forms and uses are determined by the narrower purposes of men and women; their interests and ideals shape even what counts as knowledge. Though the works of reason have lifted innumerable burdens of hunger and sorrow, they have also cast up a new world of power."
    -Paul Starr, The Social Transformation of American Medicine[176]

This is one of the most difficult questions to answer. The most cynical will point to greed, corruption, and the conflicts of interest inherent in a system that profits from the protraction and increasing expense of treatments versus cheaper, simpler, longer-term solutions. Apologists will point to tort reform, malpractice insurance regulations, and other socio-political constraints to more efficient progress.

I won't try to reconcile these points of view here, but I do hope to clearly establish that the fact that a procedure is commonly and consistently utilized is no proof of its value or safety, and that it is (unfortunately) the obligation of the consumer to do their own homework on any particular medical strategy. Either way, to imagine that medical science is some isolated entity evolving undisturbed through time is idyllic but perhaps a bit naïve. In fact, it's critical to understand that, over time, the continued perpetuation of any protocol or procedure—even a dangerous or unproven one—generates its own intrinsic momentum. This kind of technical inertia becomes increasingly more difficult to disrupt, developing a kind of immunological resistance to scientific scrutiny.

Here's a story to illustrate what I mean:

A little girl watches her mother prepare a ham for the family dinner. The mother cuts both ends off the ham and places it in the oven. "Why do you cut the ends off, Mom?" asks the girl. "Oh, we've always done it that way...ask your grandmother," says the mother. "Why do we cut the ends off the ham, Grandma?" says the girl to her grandmother. "Oh, we've just always done it that way. Ask your great grandmother, dear." "Great-grandma, why do we cut the ends off the ham?" "Oh, well, dear, you need to cut the ends off the ham, otherwise it won't fit in the oven!"

The ovens in Great-grandma's time were too small to fit a whole ham. By the time the ovens got bigger, the ritual of cutting the ham had lost its original purpose but kept its cultural momentum. We do it "because we've always done it that way."

And while today we live in an age when access to information is so vast that modern science is truly within the reach of the average citizen, we don't always subject scientific *history* to the same scrutiny as the present. Understanding the historical continuum that has led us to the present can be a key to dismantling our investment in clinical paradigms which do not serve us.

It is said that it is hard to see the picture when you are inside the frame. Medical thinkers, too, could not "see" the deeper source of the problem they sought to solve. This explains why birth outcomes were not positively impacted by the measures of DeLee and his compatriots.

Much of this failure stemmed from an almost religious faith in the power of science and medicine to solve all of humanity's problems. In the public discourse on medicine and health care, this has come to be known as "Scientism." In the case of DeLee, we have a man who was well known as fostering an unflinching belief in the potential of medicine to have this panaceatic effect. That belief led him to establish the protocols that ultimately became universalized in childbirth care. As we have discussed, the flaw of which DeLee and his contemporaries were guilty was less hubris and megalomania and more simply a lack of creativity.

De-Pathologization requires that we accept that technology and science may not be the answer to all our problems, and in fact, may be the cause of some. Returning to a respect and recognition of the innate power of nature and the body; of the compelling and uncompromising force of evolution, of which we are a manifestation, is a prerequisite to tapping the potential of our bodies and of nature, and discriminating between the technology that serves us and the technology that we serve.

To summarize:

The reality is that the primary factors for hazardous births in the centuries prior to the mid-twentieth century were social, environmental, and iatrogenic (doctor-*caused*).

The CDC states:

In 1900 in some U.S. cities, up to 30% of infants died before reaching their first birthday (1). Efforts to reduce infant mortality focused on improving environmental and living conditions in urban areas (1). Urban environmental interventions (e.g., sewage and refuse disposal and safe drinking water) played key roles in reducing infant mortality. Rising standards of living, including improvements in economic and education levels of families, helped to promote health. Declining fertility rates also contributed to reductions in infant mortality through longer spacing of children, smaller family size, and better nutritional status of mothers and infants (1). Milk pasteurization, first adopted in Chicago in 1908, contributed to the control of milkborne diseases (e.g., gastrointestinal infections) from contaminated milk supplies.[177]

There were many factors which have influenced the decreased infant and maternal mortality rates in the early 20th century; unfortunately, the factor we most commonly associate with these improvements—the movement of birth into hospitals—is not one of them. Even later improvements have been shown to have occurred against the gradient of obstetrical "advancements":

"For a time in the 1950s and 1960s, our maternal mortality rates were going down, but it has been shown that the decrease resulted from basic medical advances, such as the discovery of antibiotics and the ability to give safe blood transfusions. It was not due to the high-tech obstetric interventions, though many obstetricians are inclined to give technology credit for the improvement."
-Marsden Wagner, M.D., *Born in the USA*[178]

It is no coincidence that the historical period in which many of these factors were attenuated coincides with an improvement in childbirth outcomes.

Corsets out of fashion..1920s
Development of antibiotic and sulfa drugs 1930s
Fair Labor Standards Act...1938
US Vitamin D fortification program........................1940s
Rickets decline...1940s
Universal adoption of antisepsis in obstetrics...........1940s
Municipal sanitation of waste and water.................1940s

As I noted earlier, clean water alone has been attributed to three quarters of the infant mortality reduction, and nearly two thirds of the child mortality reduction in the U.S. The notion that birth, a wildly perilous and savage process, was saved by the technology of modern medicine is not only a fantasy, but the truth is very nearly perfectly the opposite.

CHAPTER 9
Modern Labor Practices and their Effects on Normal Delivery

Though Joseph DeLee's radical proposals for birth management were presented in the early 1900s, his legacy remains indelible. Childbirth in the United States remains a hospital procedure. While ether has been retired, it has been replaced with spinals or epidurals (in two out of every three U.S. births[179]). The lithotomy position remains standard and the surgical interventions of episiotomy (though still utilized in smaller percentages) and forceps have been replaced with the even more invasive intervention of the Cesarean section.

Today's typical pregnant American mother considers birthing outside of the hospital a radical notion. She is likely not aware that studies show birth at home managed by midwives is as safe an option, with better chances for a rewarding experience and less chances for complications. Her pregnancy is a condition that must be monitored and managed by those who treat conditions: medical doctors.

I have had many women tell me, "Thank God I was in the hospital because I had such and such complication, and thankfully the doctors were right there," But I have rarely heard a woman say, "I wonder if the reason I had those complications was because I was in the hospital."

How can modern birth practices generate the complications they so readily treat?

Lithotomy Position

We have already discussed the effect of the lithotomy position on the progress of labor. It closes off the pelvic outlet by 20% to 30%, obstructs the blood vessels and nerves that serve the pelvis and uterus, and it forces a woman to attempt to give birth against gravity. The lithotomy position activates neural signals for surrender, which is deleterious to an individual engaged in a process which arguably calls for the highest levels of self-determinism and fortitude.

External Fetal Monitoring (EFM)

Ninety-four percent of women who experienced labor in U.S. hospitals in 2005 reported using EFM, and among those, 93 percent were monitored either continuously (76 percent) or for most of the time (17 percent) during labor. Just three percent were monitored using a handheld device alone. (Declercq, et al., 2006)[180]

The external fetal monitor also never passed FDA approval. It had already been placed in nearly every maternity ward in the country when the Medical Devices Amendments were passed, which required that devices such as EFM be approved for "safety and effectiveness." It was grandfathered in.[181] So, it seems, were several other procedures.

While the idea of continuously monitoring the fetal heart rate may sound like a valuable tool, one problem is that it precludes one of the most elemental acts to promote normal labor: movement. In order for the fetus to complete its journey, it needs to spiral through the birth canal. That spiraling often requires the mother to be able to rock, twist, change position, and move in a way that allows her pelvis to accommodate those transitions. EFM makes this very difficult. The focus of her caregivers is diverted away from her to the machine. Her own focus is distracted outside of herself to the machine instead of being able to respond to the subtle internal cues that will help her facilitate the easiest, safest birth.

Systematic reviews of EFM have shown no benefit to the mother or child, other than a slight decrease in newborn seizures, with no long-term impact on the child. Risks of EFM include:

- Increased likelihood of C-section
- Increased risk of vacuum or forceps extraction
- Increased pain in birth
- Decreased ability to move
- Decreased attention to mother
- Increased risk of need for epidural anesthesia

These dangers were found for both lower-risk and higher-risk subgroups.[182]

This is a classic case of the self-fulfilling prophesy. We monitor the baby in case something goes wrong, but the monitoring causes things to go wrong, which we detect with the monitor! EFM also is often the initiating force for the notorious "cascade of interventions," the snowball effect in which one intervention leads to another, and another, all of which lead, for one in three American women, to the signature procedure for medicalized childbirth: cesarean section.

C-Section

The current U.S. C-section rate of 32.8% is not of great concern to many medical professionals. W. Benson Harer, Jr., M.D., former president of ACOG, called the C-section a "life-enhancing procedure" and vaginal birth "the most dangerous trip that any of us will ever take."[183] That C-section rates in the United States have reached epidemic proportions, then, is one of the clearest and most tragic expressions of the Handy Hammer principle imaginable. C-section represents the apex of the medicalization of birth.

Clearly, there are rare instances in which C-section is a necessary and life-saving intervention. And, in fact, the percentage of modern births in which C-section is necessary seems consistent. The World Health Organization has determined, through a thorough review of the literature, that a national C-section rate of 5% to 10% is optimal and a rate over 15% is more likely to be doing harm than good.[184] Yet the U.S. C-section rate is currently 32.8%.[185] That means that 15-20% of the C-sections performed in the US are unnecessary. That's 898,798 unnecessary surgeries.

The laissez-faire attitude that modern medicine seems to have adopted around C-sections is clearly part of the problem.

"If you really want to be one hundred percent safe, you should have your pregnancy go to thirty-nine weeks and have a scheduled C-section. That's the best we can do..."
-Mary Elizabeth Soper, M.D., obstetrician, *The Business of Baby*

While many women may have embraced the notion that a C-section is a minor surgery that spares her the pain and inconvenience of vaginal birth, many realize, too late, that the reality is quite another story. I have witnessed the impacts of this procedure on women for two decades in my practice. Extended hospital stays, chronic back pain and headaches, greater difficulty bonding with and breastfeeding the baby, and often a deep sense of loss and failure that so many women find incredibly difficult to shake.

What are the additional risks that a woman and her child take on when they are subjected to this procedure?

- Increased risk of asthma and allergies.[186] One potential mechanism for this phenomenon is that when the baby passes naturally through the birth canal, they are colonized with beneficial bacteria and cleaned of harmful bacteria.[187]
- Passage through the birth canal also helps to squeeze the amniotic fluid out of the respiratory passages of the newborn. This may explain the increased incidence of respiratory problems in babies born via C-section.[188]
- Researchers for the CDC who studied 5.7 million U.S. births found that babies born via C-section with no medical risk factors were nearly three times more likely to die within the first month of life than those born vaginally.[189]

A systematic review[190] showed short-term harm to mothers that was more likely with cesarean section also included:

- maternal death
- emergency hysterectomy
- blood clots and stroke
- surgical injury
- longer hospitalization and more likely re-hospitalization
- infection
- poor birth experience
- less early contact with babies
- intense and prolonged postpartum pain
- poor overall mental health and self-esteem
- poor overall functioning

A woman's risk of death in childbirth is as much as *four times* higher if she gives birth by C-section versus vaginally.[191] The risks of C-section extend beyond the procedure itself, because having a C-section increases the chances that ensuing pregnancies will result in C-sections as well, and the risks of second and third sections compound.

Clearly, there's a disconnect between the data on C-section and the attitude toward the procedure that doctors have embraced.

Is the C-section rate so high because women are choosing "elective" C-sections, or because women are becoming less healthy?

Evidence-Based Maternity from the Childbirth Collective reports:

"*Although many health professionals, journalists, and others have proposed that the rising cesarean rate is largely a consequence of women's requests for planned cesarean without a medical rationale, surveys of mothers themselves find that this phenomenon is very limited (Declercq et al., 2006; Kingdon, Baker, and Lavender 2006; McCourt et al., 2007). Similarly, increased genuine need for cesarean in the population of childbearing women—associated, for example, with more multiple births and childbearing among older women who are more likely to have chronic medical conditions—appears to play a limited role in recent trends, as the cesarean rate is rising for all classes of women, at all levels of risk, including those with no indicated risk at all. The increase reflects changing professional standards, with growing casual acceptance of cesarean surgery, lowered thresholds for applying traditional indications, and the appearance of new and unsupported justifications such as 'baby seems large.'*"[192]

For a brief discussion of the "too large a baby" diagnosis, see the subsection, "a+b = x?"

When I present this information in anatomy courses or professional seminars, the question is always the same: Why is such a dangerous procedure perpetuated against the gradient of evidence?

The main reason doctors themselves give for this cognitive dissonance is the simple logistics of medical malpractice. The reality for them is that performing a surgical procedure, in the eyes of a malpractice proceeding, represents a doctor who is doing everything possible to secure a safe outcome for mother and baby, regardless of whether the procedure was indicated or the optimal choice for the clinical situation.

"If a doctor performs a C-section, the perception is that the doctor did everything he could. If the baby suffers an injury in a vaginal birth, doctors believe that they will be found guilty for not anticipating the problem and performing a C-section."[193]

One obstetrician acknowledged simply, "Expediency, economics, and the fear of litigation are the three things that control pretty much every decision that's made in medicine today, especially obstetrics."

This admission may come as something of a shock to people who might associate other phrases with the ethics that control a medical doctor's decision, like the well-being of the patient, the best possible outcome, or the most well-informed and evidence-based medical decision. Sadly, these considerations are often secondary to the more urgent perceived need of the doctor to protect him or herself. The evidence of this reads in black and white—nearly a million unnecessary C-sections are performed per year in the U.S., with untold associated illness, trauma, and death as the direct result. This year, the British medical journal The Lancet estimated that in 2010, as many as 6 million unnecessary c-sections were performed worldwide.[194]

The economics of excessive intervention are difficult to ignore. C-section is the most common operating room procedure in the country and a huge financial industry for hospitals, adding thousands of dollars to the average cost of a hospital birth.

The average hospital charge in 2005 ranged from about $7,000 for an uncomplicated vaginal birth to about $16,000 for a complicated Cesarean section,[195] helping to make childbirth the most profitable "condition" treated at a hospital.

According to *The New York Times*:

Childbirth in the United States is uniquely expensive, and maternity and newborn care constitute the single biggest category of hospital payouts for most commercial insurers and state Medicaid programs. The cumulative costs of approximately four million annual births are well over $50 billion.[196]

C-section appears to be medically indicated, that is, correlating with improved outcomes for mother and baby, somewhere between five and 10 percent of the time. A recent study of nearly 17,000 home births found a rate of 5.2%, with a VBAC rate of 87%, with no increase in adverse outcomes versus hospital births.[197] Iceland has a section rate of just 14.6%, less than half that of the U.S., yet its maternal mortality rate is *five times* lower.[198] For the small percentage of mothers, the procedure is valuable and the skills of the obstetrician may be life-saving. The message we should be getting, though, is: When we fail to contextualize medicine, we begin to generate poor results very quickly.

Labor Induction

Induction is the injection of artificial hormones in order to "induce" or jump-start labor contractions. Since it is a synthetic hormone, the body does not perceive it or respond to it in the same way as to its natural analog.

Pitocin-induced labors:

- Are more likely to be longer, harder, and more painful
- Are associated with increased risks of complicated labors and deliveries, hemorrhage, and life-threatening placental rupture
- Are more likely to cause fetal distress, lower Apgar scores, and nerve damage

Jeanne Ohm, President, International Chiropractic Pediatric Association,[199] writes:

In either induced or enhanced use of pitocin, the blood supply (and therefore the oxygen source) to the uterus is greatly reduced. With naturally paced contractions, there is a time interval between contractions, allowing for the baby to be fully oxygenated before the next contraction. In induced or stimulated labor, the contractions are closer together and last for a longer time thus shortening the interval where the baby receives its oxygen supply. Reduced oxygen could have life-long consequences on the baby's brain...

It is the belief (not necessarily the practice) in the medical profession that induction should occur when the risk of continuing pregnancy presents a threat to the life of the mother or baby. These situations include: some severe diabetics, kidney disease, severe preeclampsia, severe high blood pressure, kidney disease, and an overdue pregnancy where a danger to the fetus has been proven. If induction were carried out only when these conditions were present, at most, an estimate of 3% of births would be induced.

In reality, it is estimated that 57% of American women are administered Pitocin to augment or initiate labor.[200]

Additional risks of Pitocin induction are described in *Evidence-Based Maternity Care*[201]:

Synthetic oxytocin, which is widely used to induce labor, interferes with the functioning of a woman's own oxytocin receptors (Phaneuf et al., 2000). This may adversely affect other important functions of a mother's natural oxytocin release, such as reducing postpartum hemorrhage and contributing to attachment and the establishment of breastfeeding (Buckley, 2004b).

- *Prenatal methods for estimating gestational age are imprecise and have a margin of error of up to ± two weeks (Engle, 2006), so elective labor induction will in many cases lead to delivery at an earlier gestational age than intended.*
- *Evolving understanding of normal fetal brain development has identified major changes continuing through forty-one weeks of gestation; for example, over one-third of brain volume increase takes place in the final six to eight weeks, and a five-fold increase in white matter volume occurs from thirty-five to forty-one weeks gestation. There is uncertainty about how extrauterine brain development compares to intrauterine development during similar time periods from conception (Kinney, 2006).*

- *Induction appears to increase the likelihood of cesarean in first-time mothers, when the cervix is not ready for labor and at earlier gestational ages (Kaufman, Bailit, and Grobman, 2002).*

To summarize, induction with Pitocin disrupts the mother's own oxytocin receptors and release. This hormone is critical in the early bonding periods of new life. Use of Pitocin based on due date often leads to prematurity because due dates are often wrong. And induction increases the risk of C-section, which has its own array of risks to mother and baby. How many women are fully informed of these and the other risks associated with this drug?

If induction drugs like Cytotec are used, the chances of a fatal uterine rupture increase, especially if the woman has had a previous C-section. Cytotec has been a commonly used induction drug nevertheless, despite the fact that the drug was originally approved by the FDA for use on adults with *stomach ulcers*. The risks of hazardous effects on the uterus were so clear that the manufacturer states on the label that it *should never be given to pregnant women* and there is even a silhouette of a pregnant woman with a slanted line going through it.

WARNINGS
CYTOTEC (MISOPROSTOL) ADMINISTRATION TO WOMEN WHO ARE PREGNANT CAN CAUSE ABORTION, PREMATURE BIRTH, OR BIRTH DEFECTS, UTERINE RUPTURE HAS BEEN REPORTED WHEN CYTOTEC WAS ADMINISTERED IN PREGNANT WOMEN... PATIENTS MUST BE ADVISED OF THE ABORTIFACIENT PROPERTY...

These warnings did not prevent hospitals from routine use of this drug on pregnant women, even those who had previous C-sections.[202]

$$a + b = x?$$

Usually, labor is chemically induced because the mother has "failed to progress" according to the hospital timeline. But she also may be induced, or other medical interventions may be justified based on a diagnosis called CPD or FPD.

CPD stands for Cephalopelvic Disproportion, FPD signifying basically the same thing, Fetopelvic disproportion: the baby is too big for your pelvis. While this is still quite a common medical diagnosis, to biologists, it is something of a joke.

Here's why:

In order to accurately state that one thing, say, a baby's head, is bigger than another thing, say, the mother's pelvic opening, you have to be able to accurately assess the size of each. The problem is that both of these values are variable. In fact, they are highly variable. Let's look first at the baby's head.

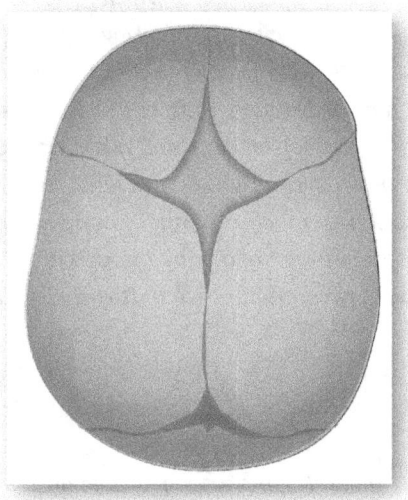

The fetal skull is made up of several soft incompletely ossified bony plates separated by masses of cartilaginous tissue called fontanels. This is an adaptation of evolution which allows for the baby's skull to compress as it passes through the birth canal. The degree of compression is, obviously, variable. So, even if you could accurately measure the size of the baby or the head, you wouldn't actually be measuring anything, because that size can and does change in the birth process. The plates can actually even overlap if necessary during birth.

Nor can the mother's side of the equation be accurately measured. The smallest opening through which the baby must pass is called the obstetric conjugate. It is the distance from the pubic symphysis to the sacral promontory.

It can be measured by hand; however this is also a measurement without scientific basis. The maternal pelvis is also variable, depending on a variety of factors. To begin with, the conjugate will change depending on the position of the mother. Lying flat on her back, for example, will close the conjugate by up to 30% versus being in a squatting position.[203] Furthermore, the obstetric conjugate, and the entire pelvis, spine, and associated soft tissues, are all subject to variations in flexibility and resilience based on a variety of factors.

For example, the pelvis is a ring of bones connected by joints. And one thing we chiropractors know is that joints can move well, or they can move poorly. When we're talking about a pregnant mother, we know that her body is under the influence of hormones like relaxin, which increases the flexibility of the pelvic joints, especially the pubic symphysis. How well the mother's pubic, sacral, and lumbar joints move will affect how much her bony pelvis can open to accept the passage of a baby. Not only that, but the soft tissues of her pelvis will also vary in flexibility depending on her state. When we are afraid or tense, our soft tissues tense up protectively. Tight tissues resist stretching. How can a doctor accurately measure how much a mother's body will be able to open, stretch, allow, or resist the movement of a baby through it?

Calculating the value of two variables is a mathematical impossibility.

$a + b = x$
find the value of x

It should come, then, as no shock that many women who are diagnosed with CPD and have a resulting C-section subsequently give birth vaginally to larger babies.

In a 1987 study published in the American Journal of Public Health, the largest percentage of women attempting VBAC had cephalopelvic disproportion or failure to progress cited as the primary indication for their initial cesarean. Of these women, 65 percent—almost two thirds—went on to have normal births; many of the babies were much larger than the baby for which the original cesarean section had been performed.[204]

Perhaps the two biggest unanswered questions about giving birth with synthetic labor inducers are the psychological effects on the mother and the baby. Michel Odent is an obstetrician who has spent a lifetime studying natural childbirth, and he has devoted much of his attention to the hormones of birth such as oxytocin. Odent believes that broad scale disruption of natural birth hormones and experiences have significant potential long-term impact, not only on the individual, but on society. He predicts that science will ultimately track down the precursors to some violent behavior in adults to traumatic birth experiences. "A revolution will occur in our vision of violence when the birth process comes to be seen as a critical period in the development of the capacity to love...Many experts believe that through partici- pating in the initiation of his own birth, the fetus may be training himself to secrete his own love hormone."

Epidural Anesthesia

Many women, raised on a fear of the pain of childbirth that borders on terror, wel- come the notion that there are medical interventions that can rescue them from that physical torture. These drugs are promoted as safe and effective, but epidurals are powerful drugs injected into the spinal cord of a pregnant woman. Epidurals have serious side effects and disrupt normal birth progress.

Labor epidurals alter the physiology of labor and increase risk for numerous adverse effects. Undesirable maternal effects include immobility, voiding difficulty, sedation, fever, hypotension, itching, longer length of the pushing phase of labor, and serious perineal tears. Undesirable fetal/newborn risks include rapid fetal heart rate, hyperbilirubinemia, increased workup for sepsis and administration of antibiotics (due to fever in mothers), and poorer performance on newborn assessment scales (Leighton and Halpern, 2002; Lieberman and O'Donoghue, 2002; Mayberry, Clemmens, and De, 2002). The spinal vari- ant of this regional analgesia method is associated with increased likelihood of brady- cardia, or abnormally low heart rate, in the fetus (Mardirosoff et al., 2002). Under some conditions—when initiated early in labor or when used with low- as opposed to high- dose synthetic oxytocin—epidural appears to be associated with increased likelihood of cesarean section (Klein, 2006; Kotaska, Klein, and Liston, 2006).

Numerous co-interventions, which may further alter the course of labor and have their own side effects, are used to monitor, prevent, and treat unintended consequences of the epidural. Continuous electronic fetal monitoring, intravenous infusions, and fre- quent blood pressure monitoring are standard precautions with epidural analgesia that would otherwise be unnecessary in healthy women. Women with an epidural are also more likely to experience bladder catheterization, synthetic oxytocin, medication for hypotension, vacuum extraction or forceps, and episiotomy. The original and cascading interventions transform normal labor into a technology-intensive experience.

-Evidence-Based Maternity Care[205]

In addition to enabling the establishment of the notorious "cascade of interventions," epidurals also add over 30% to the cost of childbirth in America.[206]

The Pathologization of Birth as expressed in the 21st century involves the application of modern technology to healthy pregnant women. Nevertheless, the birth experience of the mother in 1930 compared to 2010 bears a startling similarity:

- 95% of births still take place in hospitals.
- The use of powerful drugs in birth is still rampant, though the drugs have been refined over the years.
- Most women still give birth in the lithotomic position (57%).[207]
- Monitors and tubes all act as "restraints," preventing freedom of movement and mobility, an essential element to the facilitation of normal and healthy labor and delivery.
- Episiotomy rates are still remarkably high in many hospitals (25%).[208]
- While forceps use has gone down, driven finally by the overwhelming force of evidence against them, their use, combined with other extraction techniques developed since, from vacuum extraction to manual (Roentgen) extraction to C-section, an extreme form of extraction, constitute the overwhelming majority of American births.

After four to five generations of this treatment, women have, to a great degree, completely lost contact with what normal, natural biological birth even looks like. The last women to give birth naturally in the U.S. as part of a majority would be over 100 years old today. The continuum of birth wisdom, an unbroken oral tradition dating back to the origins of humankind, was severed in the course of one person's lifetime. One hundred million years of knowledge, power, and enlightenment extinguished in 100 years.

The institutional Pathologization of Birth—which has its own continuum that began in the U.S. with, perhaps, DeLee, and has its earliest roots possibly in 18th century Europe—remains intact. In Jennifer Margulis' book, *The Business of Baby*, she relates an interview with several obstetricians under the heading, "YOUR DOCTOR THINKS BIRTH IS AN ILLNESS":

Stuart Fishbein, M.D., thinks the problem begins in American medical schools, where students are taught to fear birth: "You are taught the model that birth is a disease or illness. Your mentors in residency are maternal-fetal medicine specialists. Many have never done a normal delivery in their entire medical career...They look at every patient is a potential problem."

The self-fulfilling prophesy of the Universal Medicalization of Normal Birth engenders a perpetuation of the *Born Broken* mentality that women continue to embrace regarding their own miraculous bodies. We expect complications, so we prepare so obsessively for them that we allow for little else to happen.

It's important, as we confront these realities, to continue to maintain context. We're not talking about a woman with gestational diabetes and pre-eclampsia going off and giving birth in the tide-pools of the Black Sea. Clearly some women will benefit greatly from the technology and clinical gifts of modern medicine in their births. To apply a natural, undisturbed-birth template to a woman who is both pregnant and ill would be committing the same error that we commit when we subject a perfectly healthy pregnant woman to the hyper-precautions of medicalized birth, painting with an almost infinitely broad brush. In both cases, failure to contextualize not only medicine but also pregnancy and health itself, results in poor outcomes. Modern obstetrics shows little evidence of contextualizing pregnancy and birth. Both have become so technologically and clinically dense that the collective angst we innately experience about so elemental a process as childbirth spills out into the media of our collective consciousness.

STAR WARS: *The Archetype of the Self-Fulfilling Prophesy*
Cultural historians and anthropologists from William Irwin Thompson to Joseph Campbell tell us that the stories of our collective paradigms, our beliefs about what the world is about and how it functions, are embedded in every aspect of our culture, from nursery rhymes to myths, from popular songs to the iconoclastic images from media and literature. Mythology is the record of the history of a culture. It is often encoded in allegory and archetypes, which transcend the fluctuations of language, fashion, and norms, allowing the history to survive temporally, while retaining relevance to its current authors and audience. This "symbologization" occurs in modern culture through any number of media, but the most pervasive myths occupy the most pervasive media.

One of the most pervasive media of our generation is film, and one of the most enduring and popular stories of our generation is the Star Wars saga. Constructed overtly from the architecture of the ancient mythology blueprint, this serial epic contains many archetypal myths that represent a psychological genealogy of our cultural evolution over the course of millennia of human existence. In making the films, writer George Lucas famously drew from Joseph Campbell's Hero With a Thousand Faces and myths and hero legends such as Grendel and Beowulf, King Arthur and Merlin, and Isis and Osiris.

The storyline revolves around an intergalactic war which affects billions of people, whole star systems of sentient beings; a political struggle and eventually a dark and sinister force emerge, which wreaks havoc on the lives of countless innocent people.

The final prequel, The Phantom Menace, reveals the source of this evil, in depicting the "creation" of the warlord Darth Vader. And how is this character generated? Well, he begins as an earnest and gifted "Jedi Knight" (language famously evocative of Arthurian legends), but is "turned" to the "dark side of the force"; he changes from good to evil. And how is he thus turned? Young Anakin Skywalker becomes obsessed with fears about the safety of his pregnant wife, Padme. It is fascinating to note that Padme's official title is "Queen Amydala," a thinly veiled reference to the amygdala. The amygdala is the part of the brain associated with emotion and memory. It is part of the limbic system, which is often referenced in childbirth literature as the key neural center for natural, normal childbirth. Its antagonist system, the frontal cortex, is characterized and stimulated by linear, analytical thinking and technology. And Queen Amydala certainly represents memory— the long lineage of tribal memory that assures her that she is safe, that her pregnancy is not a threat to her. Indeed, even her given name, Padme, is Sanskrit for "lotus," which is symbolically linked with the female genitals, and in Sanskrit represents wisdom. So Padme's name can be interpreted as "the wisdom of the woman's body."

But Anakin is beset with nightmares, which are premonitions about Padme's imminent death, in childbirth. As a "gifted" Jedi, he arrogantly assumes that his dreams are warnings of a certain future that he now must avert. In reality, his efforts to avert the danger are the sole source of the threat, and his efforts to frantically rescue his pregnant bride are the sole cause of her death, in childbirth no less.

The allegory is interesting: Medical management of childbirth is overseen by "gifted" physicians who are perpetually and notoriously obsessed with fears about potential negative birth outcomes. This fear leads them to pursue protective measures, such as external fetal monitors, amniocentesis, and a supine birth position which affords a better medical access to the vagina but has catastrophic impacts on the woman's ability to birth. As a result, the efforts on the part of the doctor to avert tragedy actually, if not directly causing them, certainly increase the chances of birth complications.

As Padme's time grows near, Anakin becomes more and more distressed. He begins to search for ways to save his wife from what he believes to be her fate, ultimately forming an alliance with a villain of absolute evil who promises fantastic powers, even the power to prevent death.

Anakin's relationship with Senator Palpatine impels him to sacrifice his own values, betray and murder those he loves most, and attempt to kill his own mentor, in order to attain these powers. It's interesting to note that the Senator's name is almost the exact spelling of "palpation," one of the cardinal clinical skills of the physician. All the evil that Anakin does, slaughtering young children in his own temple, leaving all of his colleagues and friends to be murdered by traitors, and all but killing his own beloved teacher, he does for the promise of rescuing his wife from the imagined dangers of childbirth.

Consider the incredible power of this myth, a story compelling enough to fund the generation of the most successful franchise in cinematic history, an industry in and of itself, whose influence permeates virtually every corner of the globe, featuring characters who can be recognized by nearly every person on the planet, and the core of this story, the generator of the dramatic force of this entire six-film mega-saga, the one event which drives our protagonist to fall from grace and enter the "dark side" of humanity, this one central driving force, is a man's fear about the safety of a woman in childbirth, and his willingness to do ANYTHING to avert that danger, even if it means endangering or even destroying the woman herself.

For Anakin is repeatedly warned of the threat he himself is introducing into the equation: Padme repeatedly tries to assure him that she is in no danger; his mentor, Obi Wan, also attempts to help him understand that by frantically attempting to shield Padme from danger, he is instead becoming the very source of that danger. The guru of the Star Wars universe, the voice of the collective conscious, is Yoda. Yoda has, predictably, something to say in this matter. He says, "Fear of Loss is a Path to the Dark Side."

But Anakin will not listen. He is obsessed. Ultimately, this obsession causes him to delve so deeply into the dark side that he loses all perspective except power, and treats his wife with such violence and abuse that he finally tragically guarantees the realization of his original fears.

In the symbolically powerful final denouement, we see Anakin and Padme, both in the hands of the medical technicians. Anakin is having his human parts severed in a battle with the earnest and hopeful teacher Obi-Wan, replaced with mechanical parts, just as the medical doctor's human tools of observation, palpation, and auscultation have been replaced by machines and instruments. Even his breathing is taken over by the notorious cybernetic gasping that his character will become known by.

Padme, meanwhile, appears in a scene which is so descriptive of the problems of modern obstetrics it is almost documentary. First, she is supine. That a woman in a technologically advanced universe would be giving birth in a supine position is nonsensical. That this position is depicted can only be explained by the premise that this scene is, like virtually all the others in this myth/movie, as much a subconscious expression of *our awakening collective cultural consciousness as it is simple cinematic entertainment. Padme is attended by mechanical droids who lament, "We don't know why, but we're losing her. She's lost the will to live." Except for the patient, the room is wholly void of humanity. Concerned visitor Obi-Wan is prevented from being at her side or comforting her until her fate is sealed.*

Everything about this scene is symbolic of the current, broken maternity system in America.

Here are the top 10 reasons why:

1. *The treatment and attendants are purely mechanical.*
2. *No husband is present.*
3. *Other dear friends are barred from being with the mother.*
4. *She is supine; in fact, if you look closely her pelvis is actually higher than her head. She is being asked to give birth upside-down, almost a caricature of the modern lithotomy position, a technique so counterproductive it has already been phased out of many labor wards.*
5. *She is in a fatalistic, depressed, submissive state.*
6. *She requires surgery even though there are no medical problems found.*
7. *Her pelvis is discreetly concealed in a metallic "drape," representing shame associated with the female genitalia, and reminiscent of obstetrical draping popular from the 19th century to modern times.*
8. *The aura of danger and death is inescapable.*
9. *The mother dies.*
10. *The babies are "rescued" by the technological representatives.*

Oh, and a bonus: The hero is named "OB."

Anakin's physical body represents the loss of humanity and deranged nature of the integration of technology and humanity in modern man. Darth Vader is often misinterpreted as a character who sought the power of the dark side for larger purposes, as someone who was "seduced" to the dark side by its potential for political, social, and galactic control. In fact, he only sought that power in order to save his wife from dying in childbirth. He is the doctor who sought the power of life and death. He wished so deeply to avert a perceived threat to an innocent life that he was willing to make choices that endangered countless other innocent lives, and even, especially and most certainly, the very life he sought to save. In reality, his premonitions were only his fears, not any genuine danger. The reality was that if he had trusted his wife's body, trusted the amygdala, trusted the emotion and memory of a boundless lineage of birthing women, there would have been no danger. The reality is that the only danger was the danger he introduced into the equation. He refused to listen to the clear voices of reason because he was overwhelmed with fear; he had lost the capacity to assess the "trustworthiness" of the situation and the costs of choosing the path he chose.

As we look at childbirth practices in America, we see this same "premonition," a pre-eminent fear of some imagined future. And we have seen to what degree that fear, and the actions which it inspires, become a self-fulfilling prophesy—we manifest the very dangers we seek to prevent. The tragedy in the *Star Wars* story is in the loss that is experienced by Padme and Anakin. There is so much potential in both these individuals, and in their relationship, but all of it is lost because of his fear and his refusal to listen to the people in his life who continually warned him that his following his fears to the exclusion of reality would only cause pain and suffering to those around him. The deeper tragedy is in the chain of events that is catalyzed by the self-fulfilling prophesy of doom that drives Anakin to intercede in a situation that actually held no threat.

The message of *Born Broken* pivots on the recognition that our bodies are intelligent and our management systems to support them must fully acknowledge that intelligence and integrate that knowledge if we are to foster the kind of well-being, health, and safety that is the potential of any developed society. When those we trust to care for our bodies become compelled to consider "expediency, economics, and fear of litigation" ahead of our well-being, the onus falls upon ourselves to become educated, empowered, and willing to advocate for our own health and that of our children.

The tragedy of the American childbirth paradigm is in the loss of connection, the loss of bonding, the loss of the ecstatic experience of birth, the loss of self-actualization and confidence that comes from a fully empowered birth, not to mention the loss of lives and health of women and children that occur every day in America. The deeper tragedy is in the chain of events that has led to a franchisement of industrialized, medicalized pregnancy and childbirth that not only robs women of the authentic experience of this rite of passage but institutionalizes new risks in the form of self-fulfilling prophesies of imaginary risks. This tragedy, though, is not a movie script. It is real. In this book we are exploring the real victims of this saga, and seeking to write our own new adventure with new heroes and a new ending.

De-Pathologizing pregnancy and childbirth begins with re-examining these well-established rituals of birth, reexamining their necessity and value, and re-considering the potential of the human body to perform its most basic functions safely and effectively, when placed in the right conditions.

HANDSOME IN PINK

To get an idea of how easily we can lose a sense of long-term memory, consider the gender-color assignment phenomenon. Think about how deeply and fully ingrained the assignment of pink for girls and blue for boys is in America. The concept is so embedded in our collective psyche it is not even questioned. Try to find a pink shirt for a boy or pink boys' shoes. Everything that is pink is designed for girls; everything for boys is blue or red. Period. Dress your boy in pink and you will be in for some very confused—and possibly critical—reactions. And yet did you know that the U.S. adopted its current color assignment tradition less than 70 years ago? And guess what the color assignment was before that? Pink for boys, blue for girls! If you think about it, it makes perfect sense: Pink is a soft version of red, which is a strong, aggressive, very male color. Blue was and still is associated with the Virgin Mary, and so was a perfect color for girls. In fact, before that, it was common practice to outfit boys in dresses until the age of six or seven (about the time of their first haircut). Can you guess who this charming young lady is?

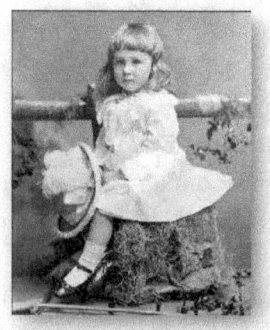

This is future U.S. president Franklin Delano Roosevelt!
But our cultural memory is so short that we have a tremendous amount of difficulty surrendering our current story about children and colors.

We encounter the same lack of long term memory in regards to birth. Our original heritage is to face birth with an attitude wholly bereft of fear or anxiety, and to experience birth as a normal process, occurring naturally at home, alone or with a supportive elder. Images such as these are so alien to us today we consider them comical.

But some see the comedy in our current birth traditions. Monty Python has a hilarious sketch in which a woman in labor is rushed into a hospital room ridiculously filled with doctors and machines, but one doctor is insistent that they also have one machine whose sole function is to "go 'PING!' "

When the mother in the sketch asks the doctor what she should do, he says patronizingly, "Nothing, dear, you're not QUALIFIED!"

The universal medicalization of healthy pregnant women is predicated by the Pathologization of Birth. Therefore, the poor outcomes that the American childbirth system generates can only be corrected by correcting our paradigm. Birth in the U.S. is technological simply because we have placed it in the hands of technicians. What else do we expect? It doesn't matter that the technology of medicine is poorly suited to monitor and manage healthy systems. Remember the Handy Hammer axiom, "When all you've got is a hammer, everything looks like a nail"? If you tell a carpenter to build a house and give him only a hammer, he will try to spread joint compound with the claw. He will try to cut a 2 X 4 by hacking at it. He will try to insert a screw by hammering it. It will not work, it will be messy, but that is the only tool he has. It is not the fault of the hammer.

Consider the obstetrician. Do any of us realistically know how brilliant and skilled one has to be in order to earn this title? The massive sacrifice, the years of study and training, the ruthless culling of potential candidates, leaving only those talented enough to work in that field, where lives hang in the balance and the complex skills of the surgeon are all that may be available to tip the scales in favor of life. Now consider this master of surgery being placed as a kind of babysitter in charge of a patient who is not sick, in no imminent danger, and in all likelihood in need of no medical intervention, rescuing, or even monitoring, beyond the occasional listening of the fetal heart, a procedure that can be adequately performed by a reasonably bright high school graduate.

If I put myself in the place of that obstetrician, I can easily imagine myself twiddling my thumbs, feeling the skills in my hands literally atrophying by the minute. I am waiting, watching, for something, anything to happen that may represent a need I can fill. Perhaps I will introduce sensors and machines that I think may detect fluctuations or signs that danger may (or may not) be present. And I can easily imagine that, at the first sign of abnormality, I might jump in with guns blazing, even if blazing guns is not quite what is called for.

It is not my fault that I, a surgical specialist whose specialty is pathological conditions which represent an imminent threat to the patient and may well require her body to be cut open, am thrust into the care of a healthy patient experiencing a perfectly normal day. Objectively speaking, I have no business being there. My talents should be focused on the patients who need me: the patients who are sick and need heroic, surgical rescuing.

We assume, with an almost religious faith, that none of these technologies would be introduced into the birth setting unless it was scientifically proven to be helpful. In reality, many of the interventions imposed on American birthing women have either failed to be proven effective, or have been explicitly shown to be harmful. Sarasvati Vedam, one of the world's foremost experts on birth, estimates that as little as 17% of all birth interventions have been shown to be safe or effective.[209]

Marsden Wagner, M.D., former director of Women's and Children's Health for the WHO, compares a few common hospital obstetric procedures to the actual scientific evidence supporting them in the chart below[210]:

Practice Vs Scientific Evidence in The United States

Procedure	Evidence-Based Approach	Practice
One continuous attendant for all labor	100%	less than 10%
Routine midwife care	80%	5 percent
Routine no food or drink	never	86%
Routine electronic fetal monitoring	none	93%
Routine IV drip	none	86%
Confined to bed during all or part of labor	no	69%
Lithotomy position near end of labor	never	nearly 100%
Episiotomy	under 20%	35%
C-section	5-10%	33%

The perpetuation of these dangerous interventions is based on the mythology of intrinsic risk and peril that pregnancy imparts to even a healthy woman. The Pathologization of Birth brings with it all the heroic measures that any other pathology might bring. And, so immersed are modern women in the toxic soup of fear and anxiety around their own births that disengaging from Pathologization is a leap of faith.

In fact, every instance that I will give of Pathologization in this book demands a similar leap of faith in order to transcend it. But I will give examples of individuals and people who have made that leap successfully, and have reaped the rewards that come from tapping into our awesome bodies' capabilities.

Taking this leap is easier when we can see that the risk we have been indoctrinated into has been exaggerated or completely fabricated, and that is the exercise of this book. Going back through the process by which we have come to these fears of our own bodies allows us the opportunity to reconsider if we were indeed *Born Broken*.

In the case of birth, transcending the belief that women's bodies are intrinsically incapable of safely accomplishing this most basic biological act is itself an act of self-determinism that thousands of women are engaged in today.

CHAPTER 10

The Modern Primitive Birth: Overcoming Fear

O f course, it is impossible to find a modern woman whose psyche has not been influenced by our modern medical version of "birth." Women are saturated in graphic images of screaming, angry, terrified women surrounded by a team of game-faced surgical specialists, focused intently on responding to the imminent emergency that the laboring woman represents.

From movies to television to magazines, newspapers, and the now gory oral tradition of women passing along the toxic legacy of violent, depersonalized hospital birth experiences, women today are inundated with reinforcements of modern medicine's primary message about birth:

Be Afraid. Be Very Afraid.

Indeed, there are few things today as terrified and disempowered as a pregnant American woman.

When my wife became pregnant, I was absolutely stunned by the non-stop exposure she had to graphic, frightening images of pain and peril. Much of this input was, ironically, from our own relatives and friends. One woman literally walked up to my wife, gazed intently into her eyes and said, "It's going to hurt. A LOT."

Despite the obvious difficulties avoiding a reinforcing of debilitating suggestions, some women still do attempt to experience the births of their native ancestors. There are many different manifestations of this endeavor, each personal to the woman herself and her own personal journey. While the specifics of the birthing plan may vary from working with a midwife, husband, partner, or alone, or in a birthing center, at home, in the ocean, or the forest, certain elements are consistent:

- The childbirth is undertaken with significant Trust in the process of birth as a normal and inherently safe event. (This in no way means, as is commonly asserted, that the participants somehow believe that nothing dangerous can possibly happen in birth, nor does it mean that there are no clear plans for those contingencies. The difference is that, in a Trust-oriented birth, the birth plan is centered on enhancing and empowering the Normal, not accommodating and preparing for the Abnormal.)
- An emphasis is placed on empowering the mother to be in touch with her own body's signs and signals, and her capacity to honor and respond to those signals.
- Labor support is, whenever possible, hands-off.
- Interventions are avoided whenever possible to the degree that they interfere with an organic unfolding of the woman's innate blueprint for birth.

These elements are not only integral to home birth, but also to any expression of the Trust paradigm. A person seeking to enhance and protect their health would begin with the premise that health is normal. An action plan would be centered around establishing the optimal conditions for health to unfold and develop. Interventions would be avoided in general, in favor of proactive, positive steps geared towards facilitating the natural process of health rather than detecting and treating the outward, superficial signs of disease.

There are many misconceptions about why a modern woman, with access to so much medical technology, would choose to forgo it in favor of a "natural" experience. Some claim that these women are intellectually vulnerable targets of an extremist "cult" that endangers women. In fact, the women who choose natural home birth tend to be far more highly educated and well informed than the average birthing woman.

Some claim that women desire to experience birth pain as a masochistic badge of honor that can be used to elevate one's status and humiliate others. The fact is that women who choose natural childbirth brave a substantial degree of social alienation and negative judgment, regardless of how easy, safe, or painless their birth ends up. With 95% of American women choosing to give birth in hospitals and most of these women having epidurals, a woman choosing a different path exposes herself to everything from ridicule to aggressive attacks of child endangerment. It is ludicrous to suggest that women would choose home birth in order to elevate their social status.

There is really only one reason the majority of women will give for giving birth at home today: They truly believe it is the safest, healthiest way for them to give birth.

Some perceive the decision to give birth away from a hospital as reckless and irresponsible, ignoring the potential risks and believing blindly that everything will be okay. Women who give birth in the hospital believe that the best way to address risk is to surround and immerse themselves in devices and technology designed to respond to that risk.

In fact, most women who choose to replicate, to some degree, primitive birth environments are not ignoring risk; they are confronting it. Women who give birth at home or in a birthing center seek to respond to risk by optimizing the internal conditions that are most likely to trigger the optimal innate physiological cascade of birth hormones and actions without disruption.

Both choices are based on faith. One choice reflects more faith in medicine and technology and less in the body. The other reflects more faith in the body and less in medicine and technology.

CHAPTER 11
The Anatomy of Natural Childbirth

Recent understandings of the human body have illuminated old wisdom. The Hippocratic corpus was punctuated with clearly holistic tenets, including the term *vix medicatrix naturae*, the healing power of nature.

Medicine has always had a difficult time with that one, and the reason is not too difficult to see. Medicine, as a field, is based on illness and disease, not healing or nature. Physicians have the greatest success when their craft is applied to situations when the "healing power of nature" is simply not enough. A "holistic" approach is unnecessary when a femoral artery is severed and the patient is bleeding to death, or a myocardial infarction has caused cardiac arrest. That is not the time to "trust" the body; it is the time to apply the Anti-Trust mentality and rescue the body.

In the longer drama of human health and wellness, and in the broader realm of normal human functions like growth, development, and reproduction, holism becomes not just an asset, but a requirement of anyone who wishes to work with and enhance the most basic elements of these processes. These processes are intrinsically, inescapably holistic: They exist in a web of interactions that include the mind, the emotions, and the spirit, no matter how you define it.

We have seen how the application of an Anti-Trust strategy in the case of childbirth has had disastrous consequences. The incompatibility of medicine and normal body functions is not only a product of the wrong tool for the job. When we look closer at the physiology of birth, we can see how the interruption of each phase of that dynamic establishes tangents and detours that have their own, often negative destinations.

In the case of reproduction, we now know that the mind, the emotions, the environment, and the nature of one's relationship to others profoundly affect the progression of the physiology of reproduction and birth.

Conditional Physiology

The modern mind has adopted an unusually fatalistic perspective on birth. It seems we believe a woman's birth is destined to proceed along certain lines regardless of the conditions in which she gives birth. This is the prerequisite for the hospital birth mentality:

"We want to be at the hospital in case anything happens..."

This is a philosophy which must necessarily ignore the question, "How much does *being* at the hospital cause the complications that hospitals treat?"

Birth is not a prerecorded tape that simply plays out once the "start" button is pushed. Every aspect of birth, in fact, is highly conditional and how it plays out is heavily dependent upon internal and external conditions. To a great degree, this is an expression of the endocrine system and the hormones of our body.

In order for a woman to give birth, she must produce and release chemicals called hormones. Hormones are chemical messengers which are sent through the bloodstream to make changes in specific body parts, called target organs. Only the target organs with special receptors for a particular hormone will be affected by that hormone. The glands that produce hormones and their target organs are called the endocrine system. The endocrine system, along with the nervous system, is a *control system* of the body. They both help regulate normal body function. Nervous system control is generally utilized for immediate, direct, short term regulation of functions like breathing, circulation, and musculoskeletal movement and adaptation. Endocrine system control, being slower and more indirect, is dedicated to more long term processes like growth, immunity, reproduction, and birth.

Perhaps the most important hormone of birth is oxytocin.

Oxytocin is a hormone produced in the hypothalamus and stored in the posterior pituitary gland, from which it is released into the body in pulses. The effects of oxytocin are a lesson in the intrinsically holistic nature of the human body, for elevated levels of oxytocin are deeply connected to human behavior and emotion.

Oxytocin is known as "the hormone of love" and is secreted naturally during sexual arousal, orgasm, labor, and breastfeeding.

Oxytocin is used to get animals in captivity to mate. Inject it into the brain of virgin or male rats, and they begin to take care of pups and behave like mothers. Oxytocin can actually *induce* maternal behavior. Oxytocin levels rise in a mother's body when she hears her baby cry. Oxytocin levels during suckling are similar to those during orgasm. Whatever aspect of love, altruism, social satisfaction, or family nurturing and bonding we explore, oxytocin is involved. Domestic fowl injected with oxytocin will begin waltzing, grabbing each others' combs, mounting, and mating within a minute of the injection. When we share a meal with good friends, oxytocin levels go up.

Oxytocin is an example of how our body chemistry and our emotions and mental state are interwoven. Not only are we dependent on oxytocin in order to experience these states, the release of oxytocin is itself dependent on several environmental factors.

The hypothalamus and posterior pituitary are part of the limbic system, an ancient part of the brain often called "neomammalian brain." It is an evolutionarily primitive part of the brain whose function is closely associated with the elemental components of a primitive living environment: danger, safety, fear, pleasure, etc.[211] It is a survival system. As such, it is natural that the primary hormone of birth is part of this system; birth could be described as the central objective to all mammalian life and the perpetuation of the species. It also represents, in evolutionary terms, a very vulnerable moment.

The Off Switch

In the primitive environment which exerted the Darwinian forces that shaped our anatomy and physiology, there is one moment in which we are more vulnerable to predators than any other: childbirth. Think about it. When we are asleep, we can wake. Urination or defecation can be arrested easily and quickly, and are relatively short events (unless you're my uncle Walter—we must get him checked...). But when a woman is giving birth, she becomes physically committed to a process that, even in the relative ease of primitive labor, may take hours. Furthermore, the product of her labor is a soft, defenseless, and highly nutritious newborn.

But evolution is not stupid. It built in a safety mechanism: The Off Switch.

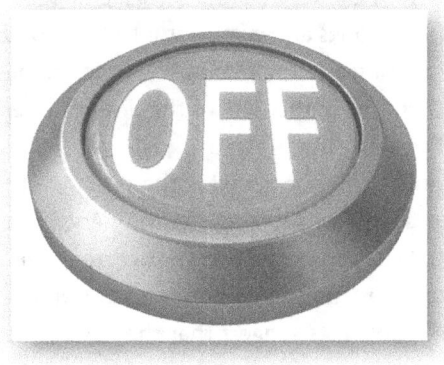

Essentially, all mammals innately seek a private, safe place to give birth. If at any time during the process they sense danger, feel fear, or detect a lack of privacy, the hormones that drive the birth process can be interrupted.

For example, a deer (a mammal with the same limbic system components and oxytocin system for birth) giving birth in a woodland environment who is intruded upon by a human while she was in the midst of delivering her fawn will experience a drastic change.. Immediately upon her awareness of the intruder, the labor will stop, the delivery will be arrested, and the deer will retreat until it feels private, safe, and alone. Immediately thereafter, labor resumes and the fawn is quickly delivered.

All mammals have similar mechanisms for birth, and humans, as the most sophisticated of all mammals, have a highly developed birth-safety-hormone mechanism The release of birth hormones is dependent upon certain external environmental conditions and internal maternal states. If those conditions or states are absent, so will oxytocin. That's The Off Switch.

It is thus a primitive precondition for normal birth that the mother feel safe, is in a private space, and that she has no fear. Yet what modern pregnant woman feels safe, at all? And as labor approaches, the feeling of danger grows and grows. In my 20 years of experience working with pregnant women, I have rarely found one who is not struggling with powerful mental images of horrific danger, pain, and death. Television, movies, and other media seem to have lost the capacity to depict childbirth as anything but perilous to the extreme. Even in a normal, healthy birth, the music and camerawork tend to be dark, ominous, and threatening.

This perpetuation of fear in and of childbirth is another classic example of a self-fulfilling prophesy.

Like most systems of the body, the limbic system has an antagonist—a complementary system which operates on an opposing physiological direction. For example, the thyroid and parathyroid glands are antagonists. One reacts to low blood calcium by liberating calcium from bones and getting it into the blood; the other responds to high blood calcium by storing it in the bones. The function of one antagonist inhibits the function of the other. The antagonist of the limbic system is the neocortex, the "new brain."

Evolutionarily younger, the neocortex is the outer part of the brain associated with logic, reason, and analytical thinking. As the neocortex is stimulated, the limbic system is inhibited. What stimulates the neocortex? Any mental process that is linear, logical, analytical, reductionist, as opposed to intuitive, creative, uninhibited, and nonlinear. Some physiologists suggest that the apex of neocortical stimulation is technology. The essence of technology is linear and analytical. Technology operates on a closed-system paradigm which is predicated by the belief that living systems can be accurately measured distinctly from their environment. Technology is logical and reductionist. A fetal monitor measures fetal heart rate on the premise that not only is the measurement accurate and relevant, but that the monitor itself is not affecting fetal heart rate. It also functions on the premise that we know what a fetal heart rate should be like at different stages of the birth process.

Primitive, mammalian birth operates on a non-logical, non-linear, open system model. Everything affects everything else, even if we can't measure it yet. The intruder in the woods means no harm to the doe, but his presence alone triggers ancient internal safety measures regardless. A chilly room stimulates the release of adrenaline from the suprarenal medulla, which inhibits the release of oxytocin, thereby inhibiting normal birth.

The modern medical birth, dominated as it is by an overwhelming presence of technology, imposes a powerful inhibiting effect on the normal production of birth-dependent hormones. And while many women choose a hospital setting for birth because they feel "safer" there, at the same time, it is hard to completely camouflage the aura of danger, fear, and peril that permeates the hospital environment. No amount of homey interior décor can fully insulate the patient from the knowledge that she is in the "sick house" where the sickest people, the most deadly germs, and the most dangerous infections are most highly concentrated.

THE SICK HOUSE

Not long ago, I had a patient, a young boy, who was diagnosed with ALL, Acute Lymphoblastic Leukemia, a potentially fatal disease which affects the immune system. I visited him regularly in the hospital to adjust him. It was clear to his parents and many of the staff that chiropractic care was helping his immune system heal and adjust to the extreme interventions he was experiencing.

Because of his weakened resistance, his room had a special ventilation system which cleaned the air coming into the room. The room had two doors: the first led to a small area with a sink. All visitors were required to wash their hands thoroughly before entering the door to his room.

On one visit, while I was chatting with the family in Oliver's room on a beautiful spring day, Oliver said he wanted to go outside.

"You can go outside," they told him. "But you're going to need to wear a surgical mask."

I thought, No kidding. This hospital is located on a busy university campus. Right outside the entrance is a landscape littered with dog poop, used condoms, not to mention the car fumes, bugs, dirt, and germs everywhere. Can I get a mask, too?

I told the nurse I understood the need for a mask out there.

She said, "No, he only needs the mask to get through the hospital."

I turned to the intern. "Wait a minute," I said. "Are you telling me that he is fine being outside, with all the bugs, dirt, germs, car pollution flying around, but to walk through the hospital, he needs a mask?"

"Yes," the nurse replied. "The germs are more concentrated in here."

"So he takes the mask off when he gets outside?"

"That's right."

Take a moment, if you will, to process this image. Here's a sick boy with a weakened immune system, and the atmosphere of the hospital is so toxic and germ-ridden that not only is his room specially insulated from it, but he must wear a mask just to get through the hospital to the outside, where he is surrounded by the entire microbiological refuse of the largest city in the state.

This image flies directly in the face of how most people think of hospitals: as clean, sanitized harbors from germs. In reality, not only are germs just as rampant in hospitals as in your own home, but unlike the germs in your home, more of the germs found in hospitals are drug resistant, and drug-resistant germs are themselves far more likely to be fatal. According to the CDC, one in twenty people hospitalized will develop a hospital-acquired infection (HAI), causing 90,000 deaths per year.[212] This is why little Oliver needed the face mask.

Now take a moment to process this next image: A perfectly healthy woman who is experiencing a normal body process is frantically rushed directly into this vortex of deadly germs and viruses; quite literally "the sick house." She and her baby are intentionally heading, not away from this place where all the sickest people and most virulent germs are, but toward it. It takes a profoundly well-entrenched programming to make that make sense.

Another way medical birth depresses natural, healthy birth hormones is by directly disrupting normal chemical reactions. The use of epidurals and other anesthetics as well as other drugs in birth inhibit the release of normal birth hormones like oxytocin.

The failure to secrete normal levels of oxytocin in labor will prevent normal labor from occurring. The medical response to this situation is to try to substitute a synthetic form of oxytocin in hopes that this will have a similar effect. Pause for a moment to consider this line of thinking. We know that a normal, healthy birth is dependent on oxytocin. We know that oxytocin release is dependent upon certain internal and external environmental factors. The medical strategy is to ignore or directly antagonize those factors, then inject a man-made version of the hormones we have inhibited.

If you're reading this and thinking, "Wow, the way you've described how hormones work, they would have to induce just about every birth in America!" Well, you're right, they would and in fact that is precisely what happens.

We know from our previous section that routine use of artificial labor-inducing drugs increase risk to mother and baby. By altering the conditions of normal labor, in this case the altering of the conditions upon which the release of birth-dependent hormones depend, we establish a new trajectory of birth outcomes. This can become a slippery slope, a cascade of causes and effects, all driving the outcomes of births towards a series of very limited end points, all of which lend themselves to the appearance of their own legitimacy. Thank god the doctors were there because we had this complication, rather than, perhaps we had this complication because the doctors were there.

The universal adoption of these methods also creates a deeper chasm between our experience and references of birth and the broken continuum of normal biological birth. And we have only discussed a fraction of the myriad of medical interventions and procedures, which disturb and disrupt normal birth physiology, like the lithotomy position, fetal monitoring, the hospital environment, chemical induction, unnecessary anesthetics and other medications, bed confinement, episiotomy, manual extraction techniques and C-sections.

Additional factors include:

- Fear. The presiding fear which the medical paradigm of birth embodies imposes a depression of normal birth hormones. Fear chemicals, such as adrenaline and noradrenaline, are hormonal antagonists to Easy Birth chemicals such as oxytocin. Fear also engages the fear-tension-pain cascade, in which anxiety generates muscle tension, which lowers the pain threshold; increased pain generates more fear, and more tension, etc. Increased muscle tension also interferes with the optimal flexibility of the perineum and pelvic tissues, which increases the risk of fetal malpositioning and birth complications, as well as pelvic floor damage.

- Lack of privacy. All mammals seek privacy when giving birth; the hospital environment is the ultimate antagonist to that biological expectation: intensely public, brightly lit, highly exposed, and usually populated by a cast of strangers, often to the displacement of familiar friends, family, or partners. This lack of privacy suppresses the hormones that trigger normal, safe birth.
- IV. It is standard in many hospitals for an expectant mother to have an IV placed in her arm in case any drugs are needed during labor. But this "precaution" actually acts as a stimulus for the complications they anticipate. By hindering the mother's mobility, they prevent her from following the signs and signals her body is giving her to move in a way that accommodates the normal progression of her labor, thus promoting complications.
- Denial of food and drink until birth. This may be part of a hospital protocol. If so, it may be in order to make the delivery of certain anesthesias more effective. However, the routine denial of food and drink to laboring women is something akin to hosting a marathon and eliminating all the water stations. It increases the likelihood that complications will arise.

Medical doctors have a high level of experience in this thing called "hospital birth." Hospital birth, however, is not "real" birth. It is a separate and distinct biological tangent, largely created by the philosophy and paradigm of medicine itself. Normal biological circuits are severed, normal hormonal secretions are interrupted, and normal psychological, emotional, and physical states are aborted.

"By medicalizing birth, i.e., separating a woman from her own environment and surrounding her with strange people using strange machines to do strange things to her in an effort to assist her (and some of this may occasionally be necessary), the woman's state of mind and body is so altered that her ways of carrying through this intimate act must also be altered and the state of the baby born must equally be altered. The result is that it is no longer possible to know what births would have been like before these manipulations. Most health care providers no longer know what "non-medicalized" birth is. This is an overwhelmingly important issue.

Almost all women in most developed countries give birth in hospitals, leaving the providers of the birth services with no genuine yardstick against which to measure their care. What is the range of length of safe labor? What is the true (i.e., absolute minimum) incidence of respiratory distress syndrome of newborn

babies? What is the incidence of tears of the tissues surrounding the vaginal opening if the tissues are not first cut? What is the incidence of depression in women after "non-medicalized" birth? The answer to these and many more questions is the same: No one knows. The entire modern obstetric and neonatology literature is essentially based on observations of medicalized birth."
   -Marsen Wagner, WHO 1985

Sociologist Barbara Katz Rothman put it this way: "It is not that birth is 'managed' the way it is because of what we know about birth; rather, what we know about birth has been determined by the way it is managed."[213] An intelligent discussion about birth must first accept that "normal birth" and "medical birth" are two different topics. If we wish to explore "normal birth," we must first establish and maintain the conditions for normal birth physiology.

CHAPTER 12

Undisturbed Birth

One of the most fascinating developments in our understanding of "normal" birth is the concept of undisturbed birth. It seems that one of the evolutionary prerequisites to normal birth is an awareness of privacy and safety. This is a primal instinct, buried deep in our genes from millennia of birthing in open, wild places surrounded by predators and scavengers.

In the context of our exploration of normal birth, this means that a female deprived of privacy and safety will experience altered body chemistry. Her birth will not proceed normally, because the normal conditions for birth have been preempted.

Unassisted Childbirth

Some of the most controversial figures in the home birth movement are the Unassisted Childbirth advocates, or "freebirthers." These women and their partners prefer to forgo *any* labor support or intervention, including the presence of a midwife, except that of their partner. This movement is based on the premise that, in order for a woman to manifest the hormonal and physiological changes necessary for a safe and fulfilling birth, she needs to be in an environment in which she is wholly uninhibited and free to express her raw self and sexuality in birth. The presence of a doctor, midwife, or even a family member disrupts that sense of safety, intimacy, and lack of inhibition that facilitates not only a safe and easy birth, say freebirthers, but an "ecstatic" birth.

Naturally, freebirthers attract a tremendous amount of criticism from even liberal home birth advocates, and the position of mainstream medicine is predictably severe. At the same time, UC represents perhaps the most compelling reproduction of the primitive tribal birth experiences described earlier by Englemann. The most difficult aspect of those earlier experiences to reproduce, of course, is the psychological. Primitive women had little reason to fear birth, but modern women have been so thoroughly saturated with horrifying birth images that it is difficult to find a modern woman who is unaffected by them. And while the mainstream home birth crowd certainly represents a population which has distanced itself from that propaganda, freebirthers probably represent the most complete expression of that divorce. While proponents of freebirth defend the practice as safe, little data exists to either refute or support their claim. Much of the data on "unassisted childbirth" includes births that were *unintentionally* unassisted, i.e., women who went into labor and delivery before the assistance they planned for arrived. This, of course, eliminates the most important element of UC as a modern analog of primitive birth, and indeed contaminates the data completely. Women giving birth alone who were planning on the assistance of a midwife or the environment of a hospital are likely to be in a state of extreme anxiety and disempowerment, with a corresponding birth physiology that is the opposite of their primitive ancestors.

No solid data exists on *planned* unassisted births, so it is impossible to state unequivocally that UC birth is either safe OR unsafe. Data gathered by individuals with access to planned UC information suggest a comparable degree of safety, but the sample size is too small and the parameters of this data are anything but controlled.

What we do have, however, are the stories of women who have opted for a "DIY" (Do It Yourself) birth. While not exactly evidence-based research, these stories nevertheless carry the inviolable merit of being the first hand accounts from the actual women (and men) who experienced UC. They contribute valuable information about the relationship between the mental state of the woman and the physiology of her birth. It was in these stories that I first heard of the phenomenon of Ecstatic Birth: women achieving a state of such openness and relaxation and trust that they experience powerful waves of pleasure, even to the point of sexual climax, as they give birth.

Here are some excerpts from various DIY birth stories :

I delivered on my hands and knees after about five or six pushing contractions. Andrew (husband) had very little time to use hot compresses or the oil massage because very soon after the baby crowned, his head just came out. When Andrew told me the head was out I said, "All of it?", which seems like a funny thing to say now. Soon after that Jacob's warm, wet squirmy body was born. How I love that feeling: What relief!...There was very little bleeding with it all...

-Earlene Stover, Liberal, Kansas[214]

Angela Jule's Birth

This was my second pregnancy and like our first child, my husband and I decided to have another unassisted childbirth. This time we were hoping to have someone with us, our 2 ½ year old son, Anthony. We prepared him well for the event. We had undress rehearsals and continually educated him on what to expect.

This pregnancy was different from my first. My husband and I were more intimately connected with each other. With Anthony's birth we learned to trust in nature as we surrendered to what was a successful 30 hour labor. This time we were more physically active and did less observing and more participating. I was a lot more educated with Angela's birth. For instance, I studied the three stages of labor in depth. With Anthony, I had little knowledge of the stages. I also explored myself and was more in tune with my physical and emotional feelings. The connection to my husband was obvious as I was able to openly express exactly what I was feeling. I visualized that the baby was lying inside me and felt deeply connected with her, realizing we are two different humans although bonded together in a relationship that will never end.

Two weeks before I went into labor I was in the bathtub and I was able to feel her head internally. It was an amazing feeling knowing that I had a fully developed person inside me and that we were only separated by tissue.

We were all just waiting. On January 31ˢᵗ I woke up with a burst of energy. That evening I put my son to bed at 9:30 after reading a story to him. I got up ten minutes later and instantly felt a warm sensation in my lower back. It felt like a big hand was holding onto my tailbone. It was a familiar feeling I had during my first labor. I called my husband at work. "This could be the night," I said. I tried to lay down to get some rest but was too excited. It was now 10:00 and the sensations were getting stronger. At 10:30 the sensations inspired me to squat up against the couch. I experienced an energy that was not a contraction but very pleasurable. At the same time my husband came home and saw that I was totally tuned in with myself. We hung around downstairs for about an hour and a half, packing our picnic and gathering anything else we might need. We know that once we went upstairs to our bedroom we were not going to come back down. We then went upstairs.

Since our first labor lasted 30 hours, we took our time getting ready. I came out of the bathroom feeling things were moving along real fast and had yet to prepare our bed with plastic sheet or cover the pillows. The sensations were more strong and frequent. When the sensations came, I felt my actions were well orchestrated. At times I sat up, rocked back and forth, hummed, concentrated on connecting to my breath, and relaxed. When my husband joined me in an aroma bath, the love between us became apparent.

When we got out of the tub we went straight to the bed, I went and stayed on all fours. Michael got underneath me and we kissed and caressed each other. At times he would rub my back. We even had intercourse and were both reaching climax when I felt the baby right there. I had an urge to go to the bathroom. As I sat on the toilet, I had my first real contraction. It was big, strong, intense, and pleasurable. As I hung onto Michael's shoulders I had another one. It felt so great to just hang there and have gravity weigh me down. I had another contraction and this time actually felt the baby rapidly drop down into the birth canal. I reached down to check my progress and to my surprise felt the head right there. We walked over to the bed where I had Michael perform the perineal massage. I held back the baby's head. I did not want to rip. "Lubricate me. This baby is going to fly out," I said. On the fourth contraction the head came out. I felt this enormous build up of pressure inside. It was the water that never broke. When her head was out I could feel her kicking inside me. I know that I was building up to an ultimate climax and was anxious for the release. Another contraction came but only her arm popped out. My husband felt her neck to make sure the cord wasn't around it. As he did that, I had another contraction. Wow!

Out she came with the amniotic fluid. My husband was caught up in the emotional beauty of the whole event as I had the biggest, sexiest orgasmic release of my life. He was crying and I was panting. We looked at the clock and could not believe it was only 2:10 am. I sat up on the bed. My placenta came out right away. She immediately nursed for 20 minutes on each breast. At 4:00 am we cut the cord and by 4:30 am we were snuggled ip in bed with our precious Angela Jule between us. "Boy, does our son have a surprise to wake up to in the morning," I thought. We closed our eyes and fell asleep thinking of the miracle that we had created through an act of love that was now complete.

-Allison S.[215]

The experiencing of sexual climax during childbirth is a concept that may be almost laughably difficult for the typical modern woman to consider, yet it is a phenomenon that has been documented in many natural births, both assisted and unassisted, but seems to be more common in unassisted births. From what we have discussed concerning the hormones of childbirth and sexuality, it may be easy to see how the two processes are influenced by identical stimuli and how the physiological experience of sexuality can be a part of the hormonal pathway for birth.

A 2008 film by Debra Pascali-Bonaro documented this growing phenomenon. *Orgasmic Birth*[216] featured the stories of 11 couples who gave birth and experienced ecstasy and even sexual climax during childbirth. The mothers describe the final moments of delivery as "very passionate," "sensual," with pleasurable feelings "washing all over your whole body."

"The best kept secret, as far as I'm concerned, about childbearing is that it is a sexual experience. All we have to do is look at the hormones in play in the process—not only do we have the endorphins, but we have oxytocin, which we know as the "love hormone."
-Elizabeth Davis, CPM, Co-director, National Midwifery Institute

"And those hormones are the opposite of the adrenaline hormones which come if you are frightened or insecure or worried or any of that. It's got to be like when you make love with someone. It's got to be safe and secure and uninterrupted. And that is how you have an orgasmic birth. Because birth is sexual."
-Marsden Wagner

"I became convinced that birth, far from being a medical problem, was in fact an integral part of sexual and emotional life... Modern obstetrics knows nothing and cares less about the fact that labor, birth, and nursing are integral parts of a woman's sexual life..."
-Michel Odent, M.D., Birth Reborn

"Birth is always intimate and sexual, although the intimacy and sexuality can be masked."
-Lewis Mehl Madronna

"It's the best of orgasm. You know, the best of orgasm is that deep intimacy, it's that moment of connection, that exquisite feeling of quaking and trembling"
-Debra Pascali-Bonaro

"Ecstatic birth is mother nature's hormonal blueprint for all women. It's not just something some women can experience. Every woman during the processes of labor and birth produces peak levels of birthing hormones. What we're beginning to understand is how important the circumstances of childbirth are for whole hormonal orchestration; and many of the interventions that are commonly used in maternity care today will reduce the release of these hormones in a laboring woman's body and make the birth less ecstatic, less pleasurable, and actually less safe for themselves and the baby."
-Sarah Buckley

My wife and I researched home and hospital birth data for 7 years before getting pregnant. To us, it was clear that, as we were both healthy and she was fully cognizant of her body's ability to birth without assistance, that a home birth was the right choice for us. To be completely honest, our decision was as much a reflection of our distrust of medical management as it was a trust of a natural process. Having attended and supported many families through unassisted births, the option of doing it ourselves was much easier to consider.

As I mentioned, our greatest obstacle was others' reaction to our plans, especially medical and childbirth professionals, who all had their own "experience", and often a deep paradigm of fear from those experiences. Ultimately, those closest to us came to support us more or less entirely.

We gave birth at our home in the woods, next to the wood stove in our living room. It was a 7 hour labor, without any complications, and our son slid gently into my arms at 5 am on a Saturday morning, to the sound of waking birds and the barest hint of rising sunlight kissing the mountain ridges around us. Here is an excerpt from our birth story that was published in Mothering Magazine:

"...as for "contingencies", we had an emergency plan for this day, which was the same as our emergency plan of any other day of the week. If something bad happens, get help or get to help. It is a simple inescapable fact of life that something bad can happen at any time, not just during events like birth. In fact, we actually came to think that giving birth was one of the safest things to do of all- statistically, safer than, say, taking a shower, going to work, or driving a car (including driving a birthing woman to the hospital!). How many people do you know have a special "contingency plan" for bathing? Exactly.

Nevertheless, this birth certainly wasn't what I had imagined: I saw it beginning with long hours of mellow contractions, long walks in the country, quietly excited phone calls to friends and family, making preparations in the various rooms, filling the tub. Instead, it began with an explosion of intensity- Julieta went straight into transition labor, with contractions just seconds apart, no time to find the birth kit, make the beds, cover the floors, fill the tub, make a snack. Just holding, moaning, groaning, sweating, bleeding, crying, laughing, over and over and over again.

Finally, Julieta declared that she needed to get OUT of the tub and onto solid ground. Shortly afterward, I was on my back supporting her perineum as our child's head began to emerge into the world.

Positioned like an auto mechanic examining an oil pan, I looked at the lump of flesh that protruded from my wife's swollen labia and frowned. To this day I distinctly remember thinking,

"What the heck IS that? A head? Can't be. A toaster? An alien? A mushroom?"

What a kitchen appliance or wild fungus would be doing emerging from my spouse's genitals is a question only someone as exhausted as I would ask. For me, it was simply a matter of reassuring myself,

"No, no, not a toaster! Ha ha ha!", until the rest of the head appeared, "You see! It's a head! And not an alien head, a <u>human</u> head!"

A few pushes later, our child corkscrewed into my hands, slippery as an eel.

I held him for a few seconds.

Time stopped.

*The blackness of the night, the solitude and sleeplessness, certainty and doubt, the falling stars and rhythmic chanting of the monks, the disarray of the house, the crackling of the fire, all fused into
one indescribable moment, which can best be described as,*

"Huh?"

We had done it. Our lives had changed forever. We had just signed up for a commitment almost as long and ominous as our student loans. There is simply no way to instantly integrate this new reality. We begin by taking in the bits of reality we can immediately manage.

It is breathing.
It is beautiful.
It is slippery.

Do not drop.
What time is it?

Time slowly started up again. Julieta was sitting up and I handed our child to her. She (Juli) was a beautiful catastrophe, bloody and swollen and frazzled, beaming in triumph. I handed our child to her and gently ran my fingerpads along his spine. I felt a slight misalignment of his first neck bone and gently adjusted it. As a chiropractor who works on a lot of kids, the instinct for me to do this was automatic. Satisfied, I somehow only now thought to check on the sex of our child. A boy.

"It's a boy!" I announced.

Slowly, I became aware of footsteps padding down the stairs. Atlas had come to investigate the new commotion. He took a few tentative sniffs of the new tenant, wagged his tail lightly, and went back upstairs, obviously unimpressed. "You woke me up for that?" he seemed to grumble as he returned to bed. Some rescue dog.

Looking back I can only imagine what our experience would have been like in more traditional conditions. A transverse position would have qualified us as "high risk" and entered us into the inevitable cascade of interventions, from epidurals and fetal heart monitors to pitocin and, most likely, a caesarian section. Each intervention predicated upon the assumption of a jeopardy that we now know was, for us, simply not there, would have introduced a new danger to mother and baby.

Overall, the odds of us having a safe and rewarding experience in the hospital were hugely stacked against us. We ran a good chance of being just another statistical component of the lowest rated childbirth system in the industrialized world.

Despite the fact that our birth was, as we had assured people all along, safe, expeditious, and wholly absent of any complications, we actually still had friends and family who told us: "You were lucky".

"Luck", we would respond, "had nothing to do with it."

For us, having our baby at home was not a bold, daring statement. It was simply the most normal, natural, safe environment for us to give birth. Every aspect of our home birth was an educated, intentional decision based on our knowledge and understanding of the human body. Planning our birth was a conscious act of intelligently enhancing the safety of our birth by aligning our birth plan with her body's birthing expectations.

Giving birth together at home, without any interventions, gave my wife's body its full unhindered capacity to access all the hormones that would facilitate a safe and healthy birth outcome. Feeling relaxed and safe provided a degree of flexibility of her pelvic bones and tissues that is incomparable to any other conditions. The lighting, sounds, and temperature of the house all were carefully orchestrated to trigger her body's evolutionary mechanisms for a quick and productive labor.

Julieta's trust in her body meant that she was available for all the subtle signals her body gave her to prompt movement, changes in position, what and how much to eat or drink, and countless other decisions, all of which came clearly and immediately to her mind, and upon which we acted without question. Being alone together, naked in the total privacy of our country home, meant that we could act upon whatever the demands of the organically evolving birth process were. This would be hindered by the presence of any other person there, and that hindrance would impact our birth outcome, and in our minds, increase the chances for complications.

Giving birth together at home was a proactive decision, the easiest decision we would make as parents. Most importantly, though, the connection we established with each other and our son remains to this day, deeply forged by the wild, celestial, magical, intimate, trying, miraculous experience of opening our hearts, minds and bodies to the simple, natural act of birth."

These accounts of Primitive birth, Unassisted Childbirth, and Home Birth all have common themes: They are relatively short, easy, even enjoyable experiences which are characterized by a high level of bonding and satisfaction. They do not take place in a hospital or other medical setting because they are not considered illnesses. The women (and men) involved have successfully De-Pathologized birth and replaced the Fear of Pathologization with its complementary paradigm, Trust. The mothers do not seek medical care because they Trust the process of birth. They Trust that it is inherently safe and normal. They Trust the capacity of their bodies to accomplish this process safely and effectively. They Trust the legacy of woman birthing power that they carry in their genes. They Trust themselves, nature, women, and the power of the human body. And the results speak for themselves. Trust is not only a positive mental attitude or set of trite bromides. Trust establishes a unique and specific internal physiological state. It initiates the release of hormones which dramatically alter internal body systems. This hormonal release creates a positive feedback cascade of more changes in the system. All these changes inhibit the antagonist system, the fight or flight response, from engaging. Fully trusting one's body establishes a unique direction for outcome—it powerfully and positively impacts the actual process in which one is engaged.

Applying a Trust mentality to a TrustWorthy body process is therefore not only more congruent, it is safer and more effective. Conversely, applying an Anti-Trust mentality to a TrustWorthy process is a collision of paradigms that detours the normal birth process towards an alternate destination, the destination we have been told to take for granted as "normal" and "safe." Yet as we have seen, the more medicalized birth has become, the more dangerous it has become.

CHAPTER 13

Home Birth versus Hospital Birth: The Numbers

T rade groups like ACOG want us to ask the question, "Is home birth really safe?" This is, in fact, a question that has some vigorous data around it, and the answer may be really in the form of another question:

"Is hospital birth really safe?"

Amnesty International reports:

"Hospitalization related to pregnancy and childbirth costs some US $86 billion a year; the highest hospitalization costs of any area of medicine. Despite this, women in the USA have a greater lifetime risk of dying of pregnancy-related complications than women in 40 other countries. For example, the likelihood of a woman dying in childbirth in the USA is five times greater than in Greece, four times greater than in Germany, and three times greater than in Spain. More than two women die every day in the USA from pregnancy-related causes. Maternal deaths are only the tip of the iceberg. Severe complications that result in a woman nearly dying, known as a "near miss," increased by 25 percent between 1998 and 2005. During 2004 and 2005, 68,433 women nearly died in childbirth in the USA. More than a third of all women who give birth in the USA—1.7 million women each year—experience some type of complication that has an adverse effect on their health. African-American women are at especially high risk; they are nearly four times more likely to die of pregnancy-related complications than white women. Even for white women in the USA, however, the maternal mortality ratios are higher than for women in 24 other industrialized countries. These rates and disparities have not improved in more than 20 years." [217]

This is a very different picture than the one that has been portrayed by the medical cartel for the last 100 years: a picture of shining, clean hospitals and happy, healthy babies contrasted against ghastly images of reckless, untrained, dirty midwives and the irresponsible women who choose them. Natural childbirth advocates have been debunking this fallacy for 80 years. Maybe this book will be the last one that has to be written in defense of that truth.

The CDC confirms that there has been no decrease in maternal mortality in decades and adds that the actual number may be twice as high.[218] It may surprise the reader to discover that there are no federal requirements to report maternal deaths (though there is a strong financial disincentive for the hospital to do so). Other reasons cited by the CDC for incomplete/inaccurate maternal death data include:

- Lack of physician training in, or knowledge about, how to fill out a death certificate.
- ICD coding rules that make the cause-of-death code on a death certificate fall outside the range of conditions considered to be pregnancy-related (in ICD-9, those codes are 630–676; in ICD-10, chapter O).
- Reliance on death certificate data to estimate cause of death.
- Medical records that fail to indicate that the events leading to death began with pregnancy, especially if the death occurred during the postpartum period.
- Medical and autopsy records that cannot be located or are not available for review.

There is a wealth of data examining the relative safety of home birth, when compared to hospital birth, for normal, healthy women. As we have discussed, studies showed that outcomes for home births were superior to those of hospital births in the early 20th century, partially driven by the ongoing childbed fever epidemic, which lasted into the 1940s in the U.S. The answer to the question of whether home birth is as safe as hospital birth for "low risk" pregnancies today would seem to have been answered conclusively, repetitively, and redundantly:

- Records kept from 1969-73 in England and Wales indicate still birth rates for hospital deliveries were over THREE TIMES HIGHER than home births.[219]
- "Mehl and his colleagues (1975, 1977) reviewed the medical records of 1,146 home births attended by five home delivery services in northern California

between 1970 and 1975. No maternal deaths were noted, and the perinatal mortality rate was lower than the California average."[220]

- An unusual set of circumstances occurred in Madera County, California in the 1960s, which allowed for the comparison of midwifery, family practice, and obstetrical care across a broad spectrum of a population—high risk as well as low risk. Up until 1960, only family practitioners attended births here, a county largely comprised of poor, immigrant workers. With the help of special legislation, care for the majority (nearly 80%) of these mothers was transferred over to Certified Nurse Midwives. Immediately, birth outcomes improved, particularly prematurity and neonatal deaths. The California Medical Association sought for the termination of the funding for the *project* and arranged for the midwives to be replaced by OBGYNs. Outcomes plummeted.

Neonatal Mortality Rate – NMR, and Prematurity Rate – PR			
Birth Attendants	NMR	PR	Years
Family Practitioners	23.9%	11%	1959-1960
CNMs	10.3%	6.4%	1960-1963
OBGYNs	32.1%	9.8%	1963-1965

This is a rare opportunity to compare birth attendants caring for the *same* population in the *same* setting under the *same* conditions. The differences in outcomes cannot, thus, be explained by OBGYNs seeing a higher risk population, as is often argued.

- The Farm Study, 1971-1989
  At the time, this was the largest comparative study of home births ever published. It compared the outcomes of 1,707 women who birthed with midwives to data from the U.S. National Natality/National Fetal Mortality Survey based on:
  o Rates of perinatal death—death of a baby either during labor or right after
  o Low 5-minute Apgar scores
  o A composite index of labor complications
  o Use of assisted delivery

The Farm Midwifery Center: The Results

Pregnancy Outcomes		
Outcome	%Farm Group	%NNS/NFMS
Perinatal death	1.00	1.33
Labor-related complications	6.27	7.29
Bleeding	1.93	1.02
Labor over 24 hrs.	2.87	2.76
Birth injuries	0.23	3.34
RDS	1.41	3.65
Assisted delivery***	2.11	26.60
Cesarean section	1.46	16.46
5-min. Apgar less than 7	1.62	2.40
***Assisted delivery is use of any of the following: cesarean section, forceps, or vacuum extractor.		

The researchers concluded:

"In this study, lay midwife-attended home births appear to have been accomplished with safety comparable to that of conventional births".[221]

- Research published in 1996 in the *BMJ* found that "Healthy low risk women who wish to deliver at home have no increased risk either to themselves or to their babies."[222]
- In the five European countries with the lowest infant mortality rates, midwives preside at more than 70 percent of all births. More than half of all Dutch babies are born at home with midwives in attendance, and Holland's maternal and infant mortality rates are far lower than in the United States.[223]
- A large study published in the *BMJ*, of more than 5000 women planning home births with Certified Professional Midwives in the year 2000 in the U.S. and Canada, found that outcomes for mothers and babies were the same as for low-risk mothers giving birth in hospitals, but with a fraction of the interventions.[224] *The New York Times* reported on a similar study completed by

Britain's National Institute for Health and Care Excellence in 2014 that found the same conclusions.[225]

- o A five-year, matched cohort study published in 2009 in CMAJ compared midwife-attended planned home birth, physician-attended hospital birth, and midwife-attended hospital birth in a total of 15,000 births in Canada. Midwife-attended home births were found to have "similar or reduced rates of adverse outcomes with significantly fewer intrapartum interventions."[226]

- o A massive study published in the BJOG in 2009, of over 530,000 births in the Netherlands, compared planned home and hospital birth outcomes and found "No significant differences between home and hospital for any of the main outcomes including perinatal death."[227]

- o Researchers from the University of Copenhagen recently examined several studies of planned home birth backed up by a modern hospital system compared with planned hospital birth. A total of nearly 25,000 births from five different countries were studied. The results: There was no difference in survival rates between the babies born at home and those born in the hospital. However, there were several significant differences between the two groups. Fewer medical interventions occurred in the home birth group. Fewer home-born babies were born in poor condition. The home birth mothers were less likely to have suffered lacerations during birth. They were less likely to have had their labors induced or augmented by medications or to have had cesarean sections, forceps, or vacuum extractor deliveries. As for maternal deaths, there were none in either group.[228]

- A 2009 study published in the medical journal, *Birth*, compared maternal, neonatal, and perinatal mortality and morbidity as well as intervention rates for low-risk planned hospital births versus planned home births with midwives in Ontario, Canada. The results showed NO DIFFERENCE in mortality or risk. Additionally, the researchers noted that "...*All measures of serious maternal morbidity (mother getting sick) were lower in the planned home birth group as were rates for all interventions including cesarean section.*" C-section rates were 5.2% in the home birth group.[229]

- The World Health Organization (WHO), in analyzing data from around the world, concluded in its report, "Care in Normal Birth: A Practical Guide": "*Midwives are the most appropriate primary health care provider to be assigned to the care of normal birth.*"

- A massive study of 16,924 births in the United States showed that low-risk women who had home births had fewer rates of intervention, more natural labors, and saw no additional adverse outcomes.[230]

In research, the gold standard is the RCT, the Randomized Controlled Trial. But the *platinum* standard is the objective *review* of clinical trials and other data to synthesize the research and filter out flaws and errors. The best-known institute for this kind of research is the Cochrane Collaboration, an international non-profit research body, which publishes reviews of published research called the Cochrane Reviews. After looking at the literature on home versus hospital birth, this is what the Cochrane Collaboration concluded:

Midwife-led care was associated with several benefits for mothers and babies, and had no identified adverse effects. The main benefits were a reduction in the use of regional analgesia, with fewer episiotomies or instrumental births. Midwife-led care also increased the woman's chance of being cared for in labour by a midwife she had got to know, and the chance of feeling in <u>control</u> during labour, having a spontaneous vaginal birth, and initiating breastfeeding. Women who were randomised to receive midwife-led care were less likely to lose their baby before 24 weeks' gestation, although there were no differences in the <u>risk</u> of losing the baby after 24 weeks, or overall. In addition, babies of women who were randomised to receive midwife-led care were more likely to have a shorter length of hospital stay...

The review concluded that **"Most women should be offered midwife-led models of care,"** and that **"All countries should facilitate evidence-based integration of home-birth services for low-risk women."**[231]

This data flies directly in the face of the popular notion that home birth is somehow inherently dangerous. The fact is that for the vast majority of women, hospital birth is no safer than home birth, but is far more expensive, more likely to involve unnecessary interventions, and less likely to be a satisfactory experience for the mother and, many would argue, for the baby.

CHAPTER 14
De-Pathologized Birth: A Model

Given the data we have on the U.S. childbirth statistics overall, I'd like to propose that the arbitrary hospitalization of childbirth is having real, measurable consequences on the American public. Most importantly, these consequences are completely preventable.

The first priority for every mother is the safety of her child, then of herself. However, if home birth has proven itself to be a safe venue for childbirth, we really should be asking if it is medically, socially, and fiscally defendable to utilize the valuable, and very expensive, resource of medical care for a non-medical event.

Dr. Marsden Wagner says,

"In my vision of a better way of birth, pregnant women with no serious medical complications—80-90% of pregnant women—would be able to choose between giving birth in an out-of-hospital birth center or at home. For these low-risk women, giving birth in a hospital would not be an option because it represents a considerable unnecessary drain on the economy and, more important, because it presents serious risks to both the woman and the baby."

And virtually all childbirth reform advocates agree that, for the small percentage of high-risk women, competent and prudent medical care is the best route to ensure the health and safety of mother and child. It is important, however, to understand that childbirth for these women is dangerous because they are pregnant AND sick, not because they are sick because they are pregnant.

These two applications of birth strategies—undisturbed home birth and hospital birth—are not incompatible opposites, but merely two different tools, appropriate for distinct physiological circumstances. The problems come when one tool is used indiscriminately of the circumstances, as if the distinctions did not exist. For a type I diabetic woman with hypertension and severe clinical depression, an unassisted home birth would be a poor choice which would endanger mother and child. For a healthy woman with no serious medical problems, giving birth in a hospital introduces unnecessary risks as well.

Instituting this kind of protocol for American births—a system not unlike those utilized by virtually every other developed nation, and, more importantly, by every country that achieves better birth outcomes than the U.S.—has multiple up sides preserving safety while reducing costs and enhancing patient satisfaction. It can be furthermore argued that instituting a system of birth in which the possibilities for maternal and family bonding are dramatically enhanced will have the potential side-effect of strengthening family bonds in the long-term, for the society and nation as a whole.

Making the transition to this type of birth will require that the medical establishment abdicate their monopoly over the birth process. This change may not come easily, but it is likely to occur with or without the cooperation of big med and big pharm. For the first time in decades, home birth is rapidly gaining popularity. In the last 10 years, home birth rates have increased by around 50%.[232]

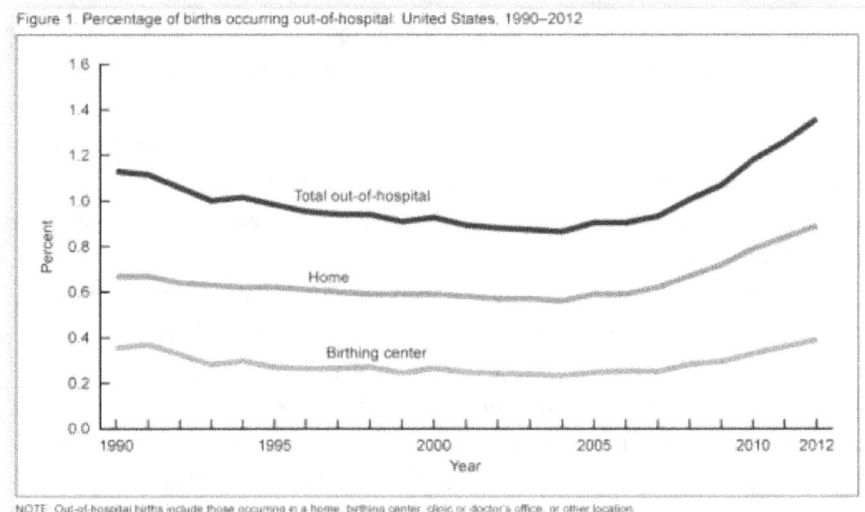

Figure 1. Percentage of births occurring out-of-hospital: United States, 1990–2012

NOTE: Out-of-hospital births include those occurring in a home, birthing center, clinic or doctor's office, or other location.
SOURCE: CDC/NCHS, National Vital Statistics System, birth certificate data.

The tide change in birth may be driven by the debunking of the mythology of birth with which we opened this section:

- Myth: Birth was perilous and deadly until it was moved to the hospital.
  Reality: Birth is a normal, natural process that was imperiled by hospitals and doctors as much as any other factor.
- Myth: Birth is still very dangerous.
  Reality: For healthy women, birth does not represent an imminent danger to themselves or their babies.
- Myth: Birth is pathological.
  Reality: Birth is a normal part of human anatomy and physiology, and has been honed and perfected over millennia by the ruthless force of evolution.
- Myth: Birth today is best and normal and safest in hospitals.
  Reality: Hospitals are likely one of the worst possible places for a healthy pregnant woman to give birth.
- Myth: Doctors are the best attendants for birth.
  Reality: Evidence overwhelmingly supports the fact that doctors are only the best attendants for the 3% to 5% of births that have entered the realm of pathology.
- Myth: Home birth is more dangerous.
  Reality: The data shows that home birth is no more dangerous for a healthy pregnancy, and even many higher-risk pregnancies, than hospital birth.

There is, of course, an irreplaceable role of medicine in birth, for those few births which require medical attention and intervention. The benefit to society of restricting medical management of birth to those that demonstrate indications for its need are vast and vastly overdue.

At the heart of this kind of reform is a long overdue acknowledgement of the body's innate intelligence—its intrinsic wisdom. This refers not only to our physiology, like the remarkable cascade of birth hormones and how their link to psycho-emotional states helps protect us and our offspring. It also refers to our anatomy, our very structure, as in the way the umbilical cord is precisely long enough for a newborn baby to suckle at the breast and incite the positive feedback loop that catalyzes the safe detachment delivery of the placenta.

In Chiropractic, we honor this innate intelligence and have integrated a respect for it into the very fabric of our philosophy, art, and science. We see the "innate" manifested in thousands of ways and moments in our lives and those of our patients. Living a life attuned to the requirements, requests, and manifestations of our body's wisdom is at the heart of a world view in which Pathologization is fully dispelled and our resources are re-allocated more towards accentuating the positive than seeking out and eliminating the negative.

Part Three
Other Hammered Items

Introduction

De-Pathologizing pregnancy and birth centers around an acknowledgment of the innate intelligence of our bodies. It is a polar shift, a realignment of alliances—specifically from outer-focused to inner. Shifting alliances represent a shift in the recognized source of power and authority, also from outer to inner. Aligning ourselves with our innate intelligence and making our health and wellness decisions with that alignment can change everything.

In the next few chapters, I'll discuss other "victims" of Pathologization, other ways in which normal body parts or processes have become inadvertently re-framed as abnormal or dangerous. As is the case with pregnancy and childbirth, the driving force behind the continued Pathologization is typically cultural, while the driving force of De-Pathologization is science, data, and evidence.

CHAPTER 15
You Give Me Fever

When I was growing up, almost any fever was a cause for some alarm, and every fever was considered a sign of being sick. We were given images of "frying your brain" if your fever got too high. But is fever actually abnormal? And, how high does a fever have to get before you begin to damage your brain?

In reality, fever is not only normal, but one of our body's most powerful healing faculties. According to American Academy of Pediatrics (AAP), fevers turn on the body's immune system and help the body fight infection. They are one of the body's protective mechanisms.[233] Here is an inside look at what happens in order for our body to create a fever (the following information and quotes are courtesy of the AAP):

A fever is usually a response to a microbial imbalance—some virus or bug that has gained a slight edge in the balance of power inside our body—and the normal, subtle immunological responses have not been enough to restore balance. News of the scales tipping gets to a central command center in our brain called the hypothalamus. The hypothalamus then essentially does the equivalent of walking over to the thermostat and turning it up. Chemicals called pyrokines are released which, simply put, make the body hot. Worth noting here is that this is a sophisticated physiological process, which requires an intentional adjustment on the part of the most highly informed part of our brain.

Here is a short list of the amazing healing capacities of fever:

- The high temperature kills bugs. Even Staphylococcus Aureus, (the "staph infection" bug) has a maximum tolerance of 104°.
- The increased heat supercharges our immune system. Phagocytes, white blood cells that "gobble up" germs, work 20%-30% faster for every 1° increase in body temperature.

- Fever increases the need of germs for iron while simultaneously reducing its availability, effectively starving them.
- Cold chills: When we are fevering, we paradoxically feel cold. This compels us to put on extra layers of clothing, blankets, etc. Take a moment to consider how unusual this act is. Our body is tricking us into thinking we are cold, when we are actually hotter than ever. This is a very rare occurrence; usually our body works very hard just to get information to us clearly. But you might be able to see that this step is critical, because if your body did not trick you, and you felt as hot as you really were, you would be stripping off layers and jumping into a cold creek to cool off. This would erase all the work and benefit of the fever.
- Lethargy, achiness: This compels you to not expend energy moving around, which liberates energy for your body to conduct its healing process.

How high is too high? Not long ago, I had a pediatric case in which the child, about five years old, who was brought in for care was just coming off a round of antibiotics. The reason the mother gave was that she had a fever that got "high." When I asked how high, the mother said, "over 102." In fact, technically, a fever does not even qualify as a "high grade" fever until it is over 104 degrees! Below that, you have a "normal fever."

Johns Hopkins Children's Hospital says, "Fever is one of the good guys. Normal fevers between 100° and 104° F (37.8° - 40° C) are actually good for sick children."

Other myths about fever include:

MYTH: You can easily get a fever that will cause brain damage.
FACT: "Only body temperatures above 108° F (42° C) can cause brain damage. The only way this typically can happen is if the person is trapped in a hot car and can't escape, for example."

MYTH: With treatment, fevers should come down to normal.
FACT: With treatment, fevers usually come down 2° or 3° F (1° or 1.5° C).

MYTH: If the fever doesn't come down (if you can't "break the fever"), the cause is serious.
FACT: Fevers that don't respond to fever medicine can be caused by viruses or bacteria. It doesn't relate to the seriousness of the infection.

MYTH: Once the fever comes down with medicines, it should stay down.

FACT: The fever will normally last for two or three days with most viral infections. Therefore, when the fever medicine wears off, the fever will return and need to be treated again. The fever will go away and not return once your child's body overpowers the virus (usually by the fourth day).

MYTH: Without treatment, fevers will keep going higher.

FACT: Wrong. Because the brain has a thermostat, fevers from infection usually don't go above 103° or 104° F (39.5°- 40° C). They rarely go to 105° or 106° F (40.6° or 41.1° C). While the latter are "high" fevers, they are harmless ones.

Thus we come to the answer to our question: How high is too high? The answer is, according to Johns Hopkins, over 106 degrees. Most people reading this have not only never had a fever that high, but they've never seen or touched a person with a fever that high. This speaks to our takeaway, which is that fever is normal, not pathological. It is a healthy response to an internal imbalance that restores balance very effectively. Cases of fever becoming dangerous are the exception, not the rule, and by exception we mean incredibly rare exception. Nearly all the fevers anyone will ever have in their life will likely be zero threat to their life or health and require no treatment of any kind.

When we De-Pathologize normal fevers, a whole world is opened up to us, a world in which our powerful bodies are engaged in a dazzlingly sophisticated dance of war and peace, orchestrating millions of cells into action and response, moving us back into balance and health, from the inside-out. When we lack the awareness of our body's intelligence, we seek answers and solutions outside of ourselves for our health. Understanding our own capabilities engenders a sense of responsibility to make choices which enable and empower that inner capacity, in the same way that a sudden realization of the value of something ordinary inspires us to care for that thing more fervently.

CHAPTER 16

Getting "Sick"

The great thing about De-Pathologizing human biology is that it's like buying a white Ford pickup truck. Once you have it, you see them all over the place. Once you start dispelling the myth of Pathologization, you begin to see evidence of the body's intelligence everywhere.

Even in what we call "sickness."

When I'm teaching in my anatomy courses, we talk about what being "sick" truly is, in the context of the immune system. Our immune system can be broken down into two parts: the specific and non-specific. Our specific immune system refers to special cells called B and T lymphocytes, which are white blood cells, which can target specific protein markers on the membrane of pathogenic cells. They can launch an attack specialized to that particular type of cell.

Can you feel your B cells working right now? How about your T cells? Probably not. But they are in fact constantly at work. Sometimes, though, they need help. That's where the nonspecific immune system may come in. Things like fever, swelling, nausea, vomiting, diarrhea, sweating, are just as much a part of the immune system as T cells, but they are things we can feel. When we feel those things, we declare, "I am sick." In reality, we are simply recruiting a more conspicuous helper in healing our bodies.

Naturally, calling in the reinforcements means that the skirmish has become more serious, so there is some truth to the new designation, yet for the vast majority of most of our lives, being "sick" is a self-limiting state in which our bodies, under reasonable conditions, will restore balance without any problems whatsoever. And, in fact, the very symptoms that we use to define ourselves as sick are the same processes that are actually making us well.

It's easy to perceive those expressions of our body that are painful, or scary, or ugly, or inconvenient, as errors or glitches. Let's look at an example of a truly sick person. This section of a presentation or lecture might go something like this[234]:

Jack and Bob decide to go out for dinner. They agree on their favorite: Chinese food. But instead of Lo Mein, they end up with **ptomaine**, *food poisoning. You may have experienced food poisoning and know the symptoms: vomiting, diarrhea, fever, cold sweats, stomachache, lethargy. If you were to stop by Jack's house later that night, and saw him in this state, you would characterize him as "sick." You are basing this diagnosis on his symptoms. But if you take a moment to understand his symptoms, you may think again.*

Imagine for a moment that you are inside Jack's body. You are his Brain, in control of every internal function. Now, Jack has just ingested a deadly toxin (called staphylococcus aureus) into his stomach. What is the first thing you think you should do?

Well, you may say, let's get rid of that toxin! But how? How about ejecting it from the stomach? Can we do that? Yes, we can. It's called vomiting. Vomiting will get a lot of this toxin out. It is a remarkably complex process that scientists called the emetic reflex. It takes quite a bit of wrangling. You can't just empty the stomach, as the acids would burn a hole in your esophagus. So your small intestine dumps a small amount of its contents, which have been in turn buffered by the pancreas, into the stomach just before you throw up. The normal peristaltic contractions that move food down your throat now have to reverse, which is very difficult. In the end though, you have eliminated a lot of the poison from Jack's body.

Now here's the question: Should we put this in the "Smart" category or the "Stupid" category (or, we could call them "random versus intentional")? I will propose, since it is removing a deadly toxin from the body without any significant harm, it should go in the "Smart" column.

But the stomach only empties its contents incrementally over a period of hours. What about the poison that gets past the pyloric valve between the stomach and the small intestine? From there it's a one-way trip to the rectum and 24 long hours to absorb all that poison! What do you do?

What if you could speed up the normal contractions of the intestines to get everything through them faster? And how about alerting the large intestines to not absorb all that water back so we can dilute the toxin and facilitate faster elimination?

There's a name for what you are describing: diarrhea. The faster movement of the intestines is called hyperperistalsis, and again, it can really only happen if the body intentionally turns it on. It does it <u>on purpose</u>. In this case, we can see how beneficial it can be, helping to prevent the absorption of toxins and speed up their elimination from the body. The stomach cramps are by-products of the hyperperistalsis and vomiting.

Once again, I'll ask, Smart or Stupid? And again, I'll posit that, since it is saving your life, we ought to put it in the Smart category. Let's see our tally:

Vomiting.............................SMART
Diarrhea............................SMART
Cramps..............................SMART

How about the fever? Well, we've just described all the amazing things a fever does for you when you are fighting a bug.

There's no question which column fever goes in.

Vomiting.............................SMART
Diarrhea............................SMART
Cramps..............................SMART
Fever.................................SMART

The cold sweats are courtesy of the fever response: When a person is "fevering," they usually feel not hot, but chilled. This fascinating effect creates a link to the conscious mind, which may be wholly oblivious to any internal problem all the while, to assist the body by shivering, which increases body heat, and pulling on a sweatshirt or blanket, which also enhance temperature increases. Smart, yes?

Vomiting.............................SMART
Diarrhea............................SMART
Cramps..............................SMART
Fever.................................SMART
Cold Sweats.......................SMART
Chills................................SMART

Now, when your body is going through all that trouble to deal with this poison you dumped into it, does it make sense for you to expend a bunch of energy on an afternoon jog or tennis match? No. So at this moment you feel lethargic. You don't want to walk to the living room, no less run to the gym. This conserves energy for your body to have available for all these miraculous healing and potentially life-saving internal events. Smart again.

```
Vomiting..............................SMART
Diarrhea..............................SMART
Cramps................................SMART
Fever...................................SMART
Cold Sweats.......................SMART
Chills..................................SMART
Lethargy.............................SMART
```

So, where does this leave us? It leaves us here: All of the symptoms that we used to describe Jack as "sick," were actually intelligent, appropriate, safe, automatic, effective healing activities. In other words, it is exactly how a healthy body SHOULD respond to a bunch of poison dumped into it. It is uncomfortable, inconvenient, ugly. But it is NOT "sick." It is not representative of a body that is failing on any level to function normally or optimally.

In this case, symptoms are not a sign of sickness; they are a sign of health.

What about Bob? Well, let's say Bob's body is out of whack to start with. He begins to feel the nausea of the emetic reflex, but suppresses it with over the counter medication. His endocrine system is not working right, so he can't produce interleukin, the hormone that tells the hypothalamus to create a fever. The medication also prevents the diarrhea that would dilute and remove the toxin from his body. Bob, however, feels fine; he has no symptoms. If you were to visit him, you might find him on the couch eating popcorn and watching, Saving Private Ryan on DVD, happy as a clam. You might, furthermore, describe Bob as "well," even though the reality is that he is infested with a dangerous toxin, which can now proliferate in his defenseless body.

The next morning, Jack is feeling fine but when you go to visit Bob, you discover that he is in the emergency room in critical condition. Sadly, Bob does not make it.

Here's the question for you: Who was sick? The guy who lived or the guy who died? Obviously, it was the guy who died, even though he was the one with no symptoms.

Now, it is true that diarrhea can be a sign of sickness as well, although in itself it is really just the body doing its best to rid itself of toxins and not intrinsically pathological. But if the toxins overwhelm the body's ability to discharge, then the discharging can itself become a threat. In fact, one of the top causes of death in developing countries is diarrhea. However, the actual cause is not the diarrhea, but the overwhelming virility of the bacteria, lack of clean water and food, generally poor sanitation and hygiene, poverty, and poor living conditions. To die from diarrhea is not a function of the symptom, it is a function of the conditions of the host. Diarrhea in a relatively healthy, well-nourished population like the U.S. is not an imminent threat; it's just an uncomfortable and inconvenient experience. The vast, overwhelming majority of cases are absolutely benign, self-limiting, and, in fact, normal. Even if the food you ate was not.

CHAPTER 17

Operator...Give me inflammation

Another victim of Pathologization is the process of inflammation. You can read a lot about inflammation in the news today, in medical journals, in various books on health and disease. Inflammation is the latest cause celebre, the latest culprit to be implicated in the causation of various diseases, including the big two: cancer and heart disease.

First, it's important to understand that there are two kinds of inflammation: chronic and acute. The first is long standing and persistent, the second is temporary. It is absolutely true that chronic and pathological inflammation has recently been implicated in many organic disturbances of human health, from rheumatoid arthritis and lupus to cancer. Excess inflammation is usually caused by lifestyle abnormalities such as poor diet and stress. But did you know that inflammation itself is actually not only a normal body function, but an extremely sophisticated and critically important one?

Boyd's textbook of Pathology has a chapter on Inflammation. It is Chapter 2, very early in the book, and the title is not just "Inflammation," but "Inflammation and Repair." That's because the two processes are inextricably interwoven.

To understand inflammation in the context of healing, let's take a real world example that a lot of people can relate to. Imagine you are going for a walk down the street and as you go to step off the curb, you misjudge the height of the curb and sprain your ankle. Your immediate experience is, of course, pain. Within minutes, you will notice your ankle starting to become red, hot, and swollen. It will be hard to move, and putting weight on it will be extremely painful. You are experiencing the four cardinal signs of inflammation: redness, heat, swelling, and pain (originally named in Latin: *rubor, calor, dolor, tumor*).

In my anatomy courses, I show this photo of a badly sprained ankle:

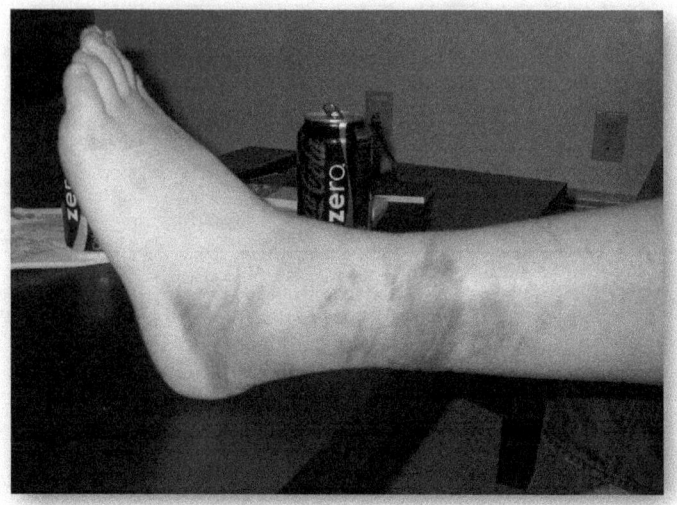

And I pose the following question to the class: "What is wrong with this ankle?"

The answers I typically get have become predicable: "it's swollen," "it's bruised," "it hurts," "it doesn't work right," "he can't stand on it," etc. In other words, we call what we see the problem.

In fact, none of these answers are what is wrong with this ankle. What is wrong with this ankle is quite simple: There are stretched or torn ligaments and tendons in it. Furthermore, those things listed above are in fact what is RIGHT with this ankle, as you will see.

Being clear about what is wrong and right in the body is critical if we are to make intelligent decisions about how to treat it.

Many of us know what the standard treatment protocol is for an ankle sprain, or at least parts of it. Most people know that they are supposed to ice it and elevate it. The full treatment protocol is commonly known as "RICE": rest, ice, compression, and elevation.

The direct effect and intention of RICE is to reduce inflammation. Implicit to this protocol is the presumption that inflammation is bad for you, that removing the swelling will somehow aid the healing process. In other words, we have adopted this idea that the "swelling" of a swollen ankle is the pathology. But is this truly the case? Let's take a look at the actual nature of inflammation, not from the popular medical perspective, but from the biological perspective.

The chapter on inflammation in Boyd's textbook of pathology is titled, "Inflammation and Repair." This title suggests the degree to which our perception of inflammation is inconsistent with the reality of what is actually happening in our bodies. An excerpt from this chapter says it all:

"In 1793, the Scottish surgeon John Hunter noted what is now considered an obvious fact: that inflammation is not a disease but a nonspecific response that has a 'salutary' [healing] effect on its host."

When you are laying on your couch icing your ankle you are treating yourself as if the swelling were the problem, but in fact it is the opposite: The problem is that when you stepped off the curb, you damaged tendons and ligaments in your ankle. The swelling (and pain, redness, and heat) are all part of an elegant, highly sophisticated and incredibly effective solution. Inflammation, as was discovered more than two centuries ago, is not abnormal. It is a repair function, and every component of inflammation has a part in the repair of the damaged tissue. Let's take a look at what is happening inside that swollen ankle.

The pathology textbook begins its chapter on inflammation with these words:

"Inflammation is best defined as the reaction of vascularized tissue to local injury."

The key word here is "reaction." Inflammation is not a random function. It is a reaction. But to what? To injury. So, we define the PROBLEM as damaged tissue (in a way the problem is you, not looking where you were going), and the SOLUTION as inflammation.

Our textbook goes on to describe the specific effects of inflammation:

"The inflammatory response is closely intertwined with the process of repair. Inflammation serves to destroy, dilute, or wall off the injurious agent, but in turn sets into motion a complex series of events that, as far as possible, heal and reconstitute the damaged tissue...."

So, that swelling in your ankle is not random or meaningless. Ultimately it is a reconstructive process that is working to repair the damage there. How does swelling repair a sprained ankle?

Each of the cardinal signs of inflammation can be traced to a specific element of the repair process. For example, *tumor*, or swelling, is the result of a complex series of events in which the white blood cells which race through your arteries and veins are slowed down by proteins called *cellular adhesion molecules*.

These "CAMs" help attract the leukocytes to the vessel wall. This occurs as the rest of the bloodstream rushes past, akin to a swimmer muscling his way across the current of a raging river (in your body, moving at 2500 micrometers per second) to get to the bank. This image highlights the amount of effort the body makes to create a process like a swollen ankle. It is a very intentional event.

When the leukocytes reach the vessel wall, they adhere to the wall in such great numbers that they form a kind of cobblestone formation, literally wallpapering the vessel wall in a phenomenon called, appropriately, pavementation. Then, in another extraordinary process, the leukocytes actually squeeze through the pores in the walls of the vessels and migrate to the site of injury, releasing chemicals along the way, which attract other leukocytes to the area. These pores are enlarged thanks to the release of chemicals like histamine, which is released from specific white blood cells in order to facilitate the movement of other white blood cells and fluid to the site of injury.

White blood cells are like the EMT's of the body. They are first responders, which assess, stabilize, treat, and communicate with the outer world for support. They have the capacity to engulf harmful bacteria and debris and protect against infection. Some white blood cells, after engulfing several bacteria, will die but will simultaneously release chemicals, which attract more to the area. Imagine a soldier single handedly taking out a battalion of enemies then, in a dying effort, firing off a signal flare to direct the attack forces to the right location. The accumulation of white blood cells and plasma fluid is largely responsible for the expansion of tissue we call swelling.

In other words, your ankle is swollen because your body has just gone through massive, intentional changes in order to aggregate huge populations of healing cells into a damaged area in order to isolate the injury, prevent the spread of infection, and reconstruct the tissue.

The redness comes from increased blood flow to the area which, as we have seen, enhances healing by bringing in leukocytes.

The heat of inflammation enhances healing by speeding up the rate of enzymatic reactions. In fact, it has been estimated that every one degree of elevation in local temperature is accompanied by a 15 to 20% increase in the speed of healing.

The swelling of inflammation, as we have seen, is the central intention of the healing process.

The pain of inflammation gives up-to-date information on the status of the damage to prevent exacerbation of the injury.

What happens when you apply the RICE treatment? Well, every component of RICE (except Rest) is geared toward reversing the effects of inflammation. Compression serves to "squeeze" the fluid and white blood cells out of the area. Elevation makes it more difficult for blood to reach the area. Ice slows blood flow as well as has an analgesic effect, leaving you more vulnerable to exacerbating the injury.

"Humans owe to inflammation and repair their ability to contain injuries and heal defects. Without inflammation, infections would go unchecked, wounds would never heal, and injured organs might remain permanent, festering sores.."

So, while we have the impression that icing a sprained ankle somehow helps us heal, it is quite the opposite. It makes us feel less uncomfortable while applying a virtual tourniquet on the healing process.

The textbook for my pre-nursing anatomy class features a flow chart for inflammation. It begins with tissue damage and shows all the elements of inflammation leading to one thing: "Repair."

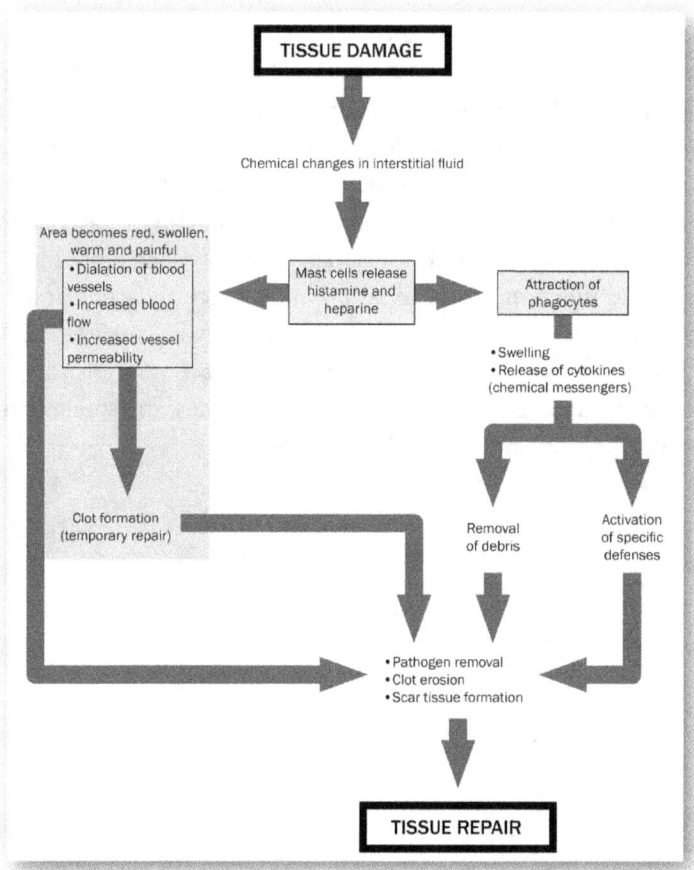

Most important in this discussion of inflammation and healing is the way in which the normal has been reframed as abnormal and universally adopted as common knowledge. But the larger problem that society is left with is the prevalent notion that the human body is intrinsically incompetent—*Born Broken*. In fact, quite the opposite is true. Every day, our bodies show us evidence of their intelligence and competence, even as we actively work against our bodies' efforts. The body does not always speak in languages that are comfortable or convenient, but for the overwhelming majority of us, we are not *Born Broken*.

The moral of this ankle story is not that you should never ice a sprained ankle. That's a personal choice that you may make for a variety of reasons, not the least of which may be that it makes it feel better. What I want every reader to get out of this story is a greater understanding of what is actually happening when you do ice your sprained ankle, that you are not facilitating healing, and in fact are impeding it. If it is still worth it for you, then you are making, perhaps for the first time, an informed decision about your body in this regard.

I can tell you that if you do not ice your ankle, it will heal nevertheless. As a runner living in Vermont, I have spent lots of time on the trails in the mountains and as a result, have suffered many ankle sprains. Throughout high school, I followed the universally accepted protocol of ice and elevation for treatment. When I learned about the healing properties of inflammation in chiropractic school, I decided to forgo the RICE method and just let my body heal sprains naturally. Incredibly, the swelling and pain receded and function was restored in pretty much the same amount of time. What I did notice was that, over time, I started spraining my ankle less and less often. My ankle had become more flexible and resilient, more resistant to sprains. Once I switched out of running shoes and into barefoot shoes, the sprains stopped altogether. But that is a story for Chapter 20.

CHAPTER 18

The Pathologization of Pain and other Symptoms

W hen a patient walks into my chiropractic office with severe low back pain, I ultimately have to inform him or her that their pain is not their problem. In fact, their pain, the thing they came to me to get rid of, is actually the best thing they have going for them at this moment.

Now, you may find that a bold and heartless statement, but I can tell you that once that person understands their symptom, they have no argument with my position.

Think about it for a moment. How does one acquire low back pain? Is it contagious? Do you slip and fall in a puddle of low back pain? Does it spill on you from an open window?

Many readers will be shocked to hear the most common initiators of low back pain reported by patients in our office:

Reaching for a piece of paper.

Coughing.

Sneezing.

Opening a drawer.

Tying a shoe.

Answering the phone.

These are the events that patients report as the last thing they did before their back "went out." But can answering the phone really cause a herniated disc? Of course not, but a closer look reveals the underlying story:

Imagine you are standing in your living room. You drop your pen. You bend over to pick it up. How do you do this? You bend right over at the waist, of course, knees straight, all the way to the ground, then you reverse it right back up again. Despite the fact that this doesn't hurt, it nevertheless is a terrible way to move. It causes micro-damage to the tendons and ligaments and muscles of your lower back. The proper way, ergonomically speaking, as many people now know, is to bend your *knees* and keep your back straight. But that takes a conscious effort, and you are in a hurry, or distracted, or you just don't care because it doesn't hurt to do it the "wrong" way. You're strong!

You repeat this movement hundreds or thousands of times a day. Sometimes you are lifting heavy objects. But more likely you are lifting a sock from the floor of a bedroom or a toy from a children's play area. In my home state of Vermont, I see hundreds of people every winter shoveling snow. And 99% of them do it in a way that is just about guaranteed to destroy their backs, eventually. Every time, every shovel, you damage your spine, but it doesn't hurt. Yet.

As your spine is getting damaged, the spongy disc which cushions the bones of your back is getting pushed and shoved and squeezed. It eventually (possibly years down the road) gets pushed against the spinal cord or its branches. Now we have a problem, because just a little pressure against these central nerve system tissues can cause big problems in the body.

Question: Assuming your body does not have the resources (mostly thanks to your poor decisions) to correct this problem, what is the best thing it can do?

Answer: Let you know you are screwing it up.

Smoke alarms save countless lives every year. Despite the fact that they are incredibly noisy and irritating (like low back pain), they are so important that they are legally required in public, commercial, and leased buildings throughout the United States.

Your low back pain is the smoke alarm in the middle of the night. Are you going to stumble over, pull out the batteries, and go back to bed? No. Are you going to seek out the services of a "Loud and Annoying Noise In the Middle of the Night" specialist? No. The smoke alarm is there to do one thing: save your life. It is designed to trigger when there is a problem. When it goes off, it is, clearly, not THE problem, but only a way of alerting you to the problem.

The low back pain of the patient who limps into my office is indeed the best thing they have going for them, because it is (finally) alerting them of a problem and the need for a solution. And just like the last particle of smoke that triggers the smoke alarm, it is typically just a small, innocuous movement that triggers the back pain.

The reason for this can be explained in the classic "straw that broke the camel's back" analogy. I must always remind my patients that it was not the reaching for the paper that blew their back out. It was the 30,000 reaches you did before that one. This is an important reality to understand because this means that, when we begin to make a correction and restore the functional capacity of the spine and back, the symptoms will often abate fairly easily and quickly. However, all we have done is remove a couple dozen straws from the camel's back. In other words, the patient is 24 straws away from another low back blowout, and 29,976 straws away from complete restoration of low back health.

Here's another example of the camel's back concept. I went to an urgent care clinic one day because I had lost all the hearing in my left ear. The ear had been problematic ever since I had a severe infection in it a few years before. The nurse who inspected it informed me that it was blocked with ear wax.

"It doesn't affect hearing at all until the last bit of eardrum is covered," she remarked. "Then, 'poof!' you can't hear at all. But until then, even if there is only a little pin point of eardrum exposed, your hearing will still be close to normal!" The body is very good at adapting, and often will do so for a long time, even while operating at a severely reduced capacity, until it reaches its breaking point, at which a sudden and severe change in function occurs.

Our current health care system leaves little room for these facts about the human body. Since we have built a health care system upon medical care, which is limited to symptom/disease equation and treatment, a patient seeking medical help for low back pain is left with the same options presented to a victim of a sudden massive trauma: drugs, radiation, or surgery. The standard medical treatment for a person with severe low back pain is anti-inflammatory drugs, muscle relaxing drugs, and painkillers. It would be hard to think of a treatment plan that more closely mirrors the "removing the battery from the smoke alarm" analogy. In my anatomy classes I call this "The Trifecta of Dysfunction." We remove the natural inflammatory reaction, which we have seen is an integral part of our body's efforts to heal and repair the damaged area. We chemically relax muscles that have tightened to protect the area while we ply the patient with pain killers. Both of these measures serve to create a false sense of repair even while the actual repair process has been thwarted. We are encouraged to use the area more, and while we are damaging our fragile bodies, we are all the while feeling fine because we have been disconnected from the natural pain signals that our body had been producing. Not only does this strategy interrupt and prolong healing, it leaves the region more susceptible to repeated injuries.

One day, shortly after we had been discussing these issues in class, a student raised her hand during a break and said,

"I had my first 'Dr. Matt Moment.' "

I had no idea what a "Dr. Matt Moment" would be and was a little afraid to ask! She continued:

"After our discussion of inflammation and healing, I went home to find that our dog was hurt. He was limping badly and couldn't put any pressure on his left front foot. So we took him to the vet. Well, they checked him out and did x-rays and tests, and they finally said they didn't know what was wrong with him. But they still prescribed…muscle relaxants, anti-inflammatories, and painkillers! 'The Trifecta of Dysfunction,' I told them! They asked what I meant and I explained how all of these measures would only suppress healing processes in his body and not help him heal. Not only that, they would mask the pain signals and encourage him to use the foot before it had actually healed! That doesn't help him fix his foot; it actually prolongs it!

So, we got into a bit of an argument and I basically told them off and took Buster home. The next day, his limp was even worse. But we just took care of him and let him keep his weight off it, and gave him time. He hobbled and limped around all day. The day after that, it seemed to be better. And the NEXT day—it was as if nothing had happened! Completely healed! And I called that vet and told him! Imagine what would have happened if we had spent all that money on all those drugs, which all have side effects, and how much longer would it have taken him to heal his foot if he had been able to walk around on it and run and jump…!"

The most important thing to understand in this story is that many people have not only been indoctrinated into equating their symptoms with sickness, but furthermore, equating the masking of symptoms with healing.

This is another problem with Pathologization. It engenders a care system which rewards short-term patch-ups instead of long-term solutions. And when it comes to the body, short-term patch-ups are much, much more expensive in the long run.

I want to describe the healing process of these patients who come to us with, say, severe chronic low back pain, because it informs our discussion of Pathologization in other ways.

The path to healing for these patients begins with chiropractic care, which addresses the deeply embedded regions of stress and tension, which have accumulated and embedded themselves in the tissues around the spine. Chiropractic will also help make sure that the patient's spine is aligned properly, otherwise stress put on the spine will be like "hammering a bent nail." We'll also begin the process of restoring full mobility to the joints of the spine so that the individual is more able to move freely and adapt to the demands they put on their body. All this will also help reduce any nerve disruption that is taking place in the spine.

We'll make sure the patient not only knows how to move in a healthier way, but that they understand that their incapacity is directly linked to whether they practice proper movement or not.

Almost always, improving the functional and structural integrity of the spine and improving the way in which the patient uses their body results in a healing of the damaged tissues and a resolution of the discomfort they are experiencing. However, I want to draw your attention to where the healing came from. It did not come from the chiropractic adjustments—those only addresses structure, function, and nerve flow. It did not come from better ergonomics as that just reduced the source of irritation and continuing stress. Where did the healing come from? It came from the body itself. In fact, the body had been "healing" all the while, even during the severe pain. As we saw in the previous section, the pain itself was a healing process, not only in that it alerted the person of the need for change, but the pain was probably at least partially from inflammation, which is a process of physical reconstruction.

These measures simply removed obstructions to that healing process expressing itself more clearly and fully. It's like having an iPod playing a symphony and then throwing a sweatshirt, then a blanket, then a pillow, then a couple of tee shirts on top of it. You may hear some muffled sounds, but it may just come across as rancor and static. As you remove the layers, the music becomes clearer and clearer, and the beauty of the song becomes more apparent. However, you would never confuse the removing of a sweatshirt from a pile of debris with playing a Mozart concerto. As long as we are alive, that symphony is playing. Our health potential is measured by the degree of interference we can prevent so that the music can reach both ourselves and the world.

Health care needs therapeutic strategies based on the ongoing assessment of functional capacity as well as a fundamental change in how the person uses their body. In this, a cycle of critical communication is completed in which the body "talked" to the person and the person responded. This "dialogue" with the body is critical because symptoms, in the body, are not only powerful warning signs, but often they are manifestations of a healing corrective force, as in inflammation.

Living De-Pathologized means looking closer at the messages our bodies give us through both pleasant and unpleasant means, as well as recognizing and facilitating the healing nature of our symptoms.

Sinusitis

In 1990, a colleague of mine, Dr. Joe Accurso, a chiropractor from Florida who recently passed away, told me the following story. That night, I couldn't sleep. It wasn't what was in the story. It's what was *not* told, what *could* have happened. What *does* happen every day, in chiropractor's offices and medical doctor's offices all over the world.

Here is the sinusitis story:

A patient comes into Dr. Joe's office with chronic sinusitis. He's got a runny nose, with inflammation in his nasal tissues; essentially, he's got an upper respiratory infection. He's miserable; he says, "Doc, you've gotta help me."

Dr. Joe says, "Well, here's what I'll do. I'll check your spine, and if I find anything out of whack, I'll correct it. That will help your whole body to work better."

The guy says, "But what about my nose?"

Dr. Joe says, "Look, this is what I do. I don't treat symptoms. I help the body work better by removing obstructions to the flow of nerve energy between your brain and your body. Maybe that'll help your nose, maybe not. Either way, I know you'll be healthier."

Well, the guy says, what have I got to lose? He gets adjusted at Dr. Joe's for a few weeks. One day he comes in and says,

"Doc, I don't know what you're doing to me, but my symptoms are ten times worse!" I mean, it was just pouring out of him.

Dr. Joe just says, "Look, I don't know about your symptoms, but your spine is doing great. The vertebrae are more aligned, they're moving better, the tension of the muscles along the spine has gone away, your short left leg has evened, your EMG readings have balanced. You can't have those things happen and NOT be healthier. Tell me again what you do for work."

"I work down at the boatyard, stripping paint off the boats."

"Okay, tell me what type of respirator you use."

Pause.

"Respirator?"

"Yes. A respirator. A mask. To protect your lungs from the dust and fumes."

Turns out the guy didn't use a respirator. In fact, he didn't use a mask of any kind. He was breathing in toxic, lead-based marine paint dust and fumes eight hours a day, six days a week. By this point in the story, most people listening are starting to have the little lightbulbs going on over their heads. What was happening was that this guy's body was responding to all the noxious dust and fumes by generating what we would call an upper respiratory tract infection. Tiny cells in his windpipe called goblet cells were turning the baloney sandwich he had for lunch into a sticky substance called mucus, which captured some of the airborne irritants. Microscopic hairs then swept the poisons upward, against gravity, where they were eventually either swallowed, coughed out, or drained through the nose.

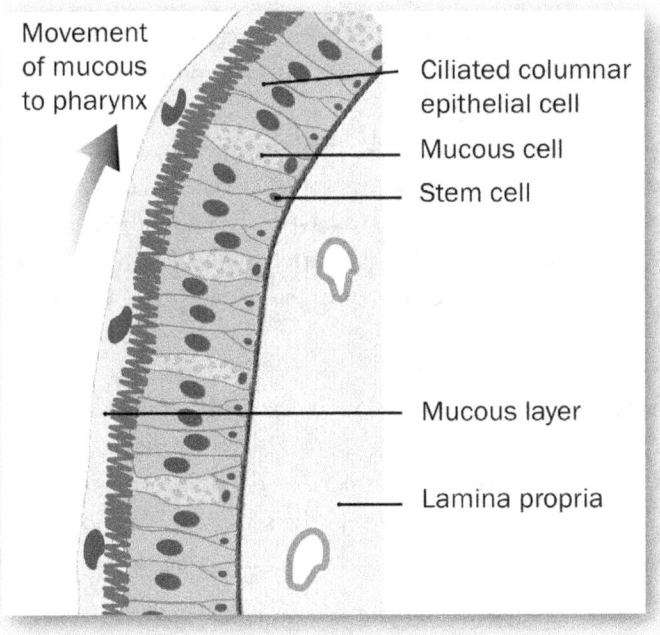

Movement of mucous to pharynx

Ciliated columnar epithelial cell

Mucous cell

Stem cell

Mucous layer

Lamina propria

So, in essence the symptom the patient presented with, sinusitis, was quite literally saving his life. It was removing toxic poisons from his air passages, and the guy didn't even know it. He thought his problem was his symptom, but in reality, his symptom was not only alerting him of an actual problem, it was also representing positive, productive steps his body was taking to ameliorate the problem.

It's easy to see, then, that the healthier his body got, in this case through chiropractic care, the better it got at creating these corrective (though uncomfortable) symptoms. In this case, more symptoms were a sign of greater health.

That's where Dr. Joe's story ended, but that's not the part of the story that kept me up that night.

That night I started thinking about what would have happened at a medical doctor's office or many chiropractic offices for that matter. The patient would have come into the office. He would be given an initial history form. That form would have, as the first diagnostic question, "What is your chief complaint?"—the "CC," as it is called.

His care, then, would have been geared toward alleviating his chief complaint. How would that have looked, I thought, if Dr. Joe was a typical chiropractor? He would have accepted him as a "sinusitis" patient, with the goal of symptomatic relief, adjusted him for a while, then, confronted with the information that the patient's symptoms had gotten worse, he would have either dismissed him from care, referred him out or altered his treatment in order to achieve a positive clinical outcome (symptomatic relief: this is called "treating the cause" in alternative circles, but it is anything but). What would have happened if he found the exact type of adjustment that generated relief for the patient? Would the patient have been satisfied? Sure. But he also would now be receiving adjustments that were turning OFF healthy nerve flow rather than enhancing it. He would have been leading the patient more comfortably toward an early grave.

This example illuminates a serious danger to basing a strategy for care on the removal of symptoms. This danger exists regardless of what field practices it, alternative or mainstream. Basing an outcome assessment on the amelioration of symptoms fails to take into consideration the potential that the symptom may not be abnormal at all. In fact, in my experience as a health care provider, I have found this to be the rule far more often than the exception.

Fortunately, there is a model we can use to avoid the pitfalls of symptom-based care. It begins with recognizing the intrinsic intelligence of the body. Interventions, rather than being oriented to masking the symptom or even correcting "the cause" of the symptom, are geared toward *responding to* the body and supporting its efforts.

Years ago, a patient came to me and said, "Doc, I have a headache. What do you think...garlic?" I paused and smiled and gave the answer I have given thousands of times in my office, "I don't know. What is your body telling you?"

It's fun to watch the reaction when I use this response. First, people are not used to their doctor saying, "I don't know." Second, they are not used to being regarded as experts on their own body. The notion that they may themselves have answers to their own questions is often simultaneously flummoxing and intriguing. This person was quiet for a moment, clearly letting the question percolate down through her mind to her heart. Then she said, with some clarity and directness, "It's telling me to go the ATM on Cherry Street, get out some cash, go to Origanum (the local health food store) and pick up some fresh whole food (none of which was garlic by the way), treat myself to a healthy meal and go to bed early."

"Interesting!" I said.

The next day I saw the patient again and asked her what she did.

"I went to the ATM on Cherry Street, got out some cash, bought some veggies at Origanum, treated myself to a healthy meal and went to bed," she responded.

And I had to ask, "And how is the headache?"

"What headache?" she replied.

You see, not only had the headache gone away, but it had also taken a back seat to the new connection and relationship this person had begun to develop with her body. In fact, as the years have gone on, I have begun to wonder how much of our suffering in our bodies is itself driven by the disconnection we maintain between our bodies and ourselves.

CHAPTER 19

The Expendables

When I was about eight years old, I underwent surgery under a general anesthetic. I clearly remember the anesthesiologist instructing me to count down from 100 as I slowly faded into oblivion, rebreathing the air I expelled into the warm plastic mouthpiece.

I was not sick.

I was a snorer.

At that time, in the late 1960s, the surgery I was having done, a tonsillectomy, was so routine that some hospitals offered two-for-one deals: Bring one kid in for the procedure and get his or her sibling cut for free. Clinically, indications for a tonsillectomy were inconsistent and, frankly, rather spurious. Surgical rates varied widely across geographical areas and diagnostic criterion were inconsistent.

"A 1937 textbook included a long laundry list of symptoms for which tonsillectomies were appropriate, including "any interference with respiration, day or night," nor had guidelines improved by the 1970s, where a qualitative study of Scottish physicians found quite different decision rules to decide who got surgery. One physician paid particular attention to inflammation near the tonsil as a reliable sign, while another ignored such inflammation but instead focused on cervical lymph nodes in the neck.
- Handbook of Health Economics Vol 2, edited by Mark
V. Pauly, Thomas G. McGuire, Pedro Pita Barros

With tonsillectomy rates in the U.S. soaring during the 1960s, it became more difficult to scientifically justify the procedure on any diagnostic scale. Dr. John Wennberg from the Dartmouth School of Medicine first noticed this when he realized that if his home were located just 100 yards farther north, his children would be in a school district where 70 percent of all children received tonsillectomies. Instead, they lived in a school district where there was only a 20 percent chance that they would undergo the operation.

A 1934 study by the American Child Health Association in New York was designed to measure the overall fraction of children deemed appropriate for tonsillectomy. John Wennberg described the surprising results of the study:

"The research design required random sampling of 1,000 school children. Upon examination, 60% were found to have already undergone tonsillectomy. The remaining 40% were examined by the school physicians, who selected 45% in need of an operation. To make sure that no one in need of a tonsillectomy was left out, the Association arranged for children not selected for a tonsillectomy to be re-examined by another group of physicians. Perhaps to everyone's surprise, the second wave of physicians recommended that 40% of these have the operation. Still not content that unmet need had been adequately detected, the Association then arranged yet a third examination of the twice-rejected children by another group of physicians. On the third try, the physicians produced recommendations for the operation on 44% of the children. By the end of the three-examination process, only 65 children of the original 1,000 had not been recommended for tonsillectomy."

The possibility that, in 1934, 94% of American children were cursed with defective tonsils, and, just a few decades later, that number has dropped to less than 1%, is obviously absurd. (The current tonsillectomy "rate" is 0.53 per thousand children.)[235]

Columnist Maggie Mahar describes the Semmelveisian response of the medical community to Wennberg's data and his whistle-blowing characterization of the tonsillectomy epidemic in the medical journal *Pediatric* as a half-century long "large-scale, uncontrolled surgical experiment":

"The story of Wennberg's career also reveals how, for decades, American medicine resisted accepting Wennberg's work. "The problem is that all of this stuff is so antithetical to the dominant ideology in the medical community—so antithetical that they can't bear to talk about it," Wennberg explains. The fact that he speaks in the present tense suggests that the "dominant ideology" lingers still. But what exactly is that ideology?

"Manifest efficacy," Wennberg says, smiling. *"Everything we do [in medicine] is effective."*[236]

This term, manifest efficacy, helps but ultimately falls short of answering the most common question I get when presenting this information to groups: How do these procedures survive so vigorously for so long without any scientific backing? In the case of this procedure, justification for the surgery was ultimately simple—the tonsils were considered to be a "vestigial organ." In other words, it's a nonfunctional remnant of evolution. We now know that the tonsils are anything but vestigial. They are classified as lymphoid organs, and are considered to be a crucial immunological protector of the upper respiratory system. Lymphoid organs like the tonsils (of which we actually have five) house B and T lymphocytes, specialized white blood cells, which have unique abilities to fight off infections.

The deeper driving force behind the tonsillectomy craze was not only a tacit assumption of medical veracity; it was fueled by Pathologization. Doctors saw swollen tonsils and blamed the body.

I recently had a pop-up ad appear on my home page for an acne medication. This was the tag line:

"Blame Biology for Breakouts! Call Your Doctor—Ask about Epiduro Gel!"

Pathologization is dangerous because it engenders an abdication of personal responsibility for health while simultaneously monetizing superficial measures.

In reality, the tonsils only become swollen as they fill with more protective white blood cells; tonsillitis is, like acute inflammation, a normal reaction to some other problem in the body. Removing the tonsils will do nothing about what has caused them to react.

After my tonsils were removed, I still snored.

Pathologization, and removal of body parts, is a natural consequence of a health care system whose sole arbiter is the guy whose job it is to cut stuff out of people. Honestly, what else do we expect? The dominant thinking in medicine regarding these issues seems to have been: If we don't know what it does, it must not do anything. The balancing force to Pathologization is the Trust principle, whose counter statement is, "If we don't know what it does, it almost definitely does something, and probably something important." There may be vestigial organs, but so far every one we've identified has not only had a function, but a very, very important function. B and T cells, you see, help us fight off cancer.

But if you've had your tonsils removed, don't worry, you have another source for lymphoid organs: your appendix.

Of course, the appendix is another one of the "Expendables," or body parts we have been encouraged to believe we can do without because they not only have no function but are actually an obstruction to good health. In the introduction, I quoted Dr. Robert Acland as he narrates the human dissection videos I use in my anatomy courses: "The appendix is a vestigial but potentially troublesome organ..."[237] And while it is true that an inflamed appendix is an authentic threat to your health and life, it is equally untrue that the organ has no function and removing it has no consequence.

Martini's *Fundamentals of Anatomy & Physiology* erases any ambiguity over this question. The appendix is prominently featured under "MALT" tissues—Mucosa-Associated Lymphoid Tissue—and described as having the function of "protecting the epithelia of the digestive, respiratory, urinary and reproductive systems."[238] The walls of the appendix contain a mass of fused lymphoid nodules, which, just like the tonsils, contain B lymphocytes, T lymphocytes, and macrophages, all which are immune system cells which fight infection.

Current research suggests that not only does the appendix operate as "the breaker switch to the lower GI tract," housing lymphocytes and macrophages which protect the intestines, but it also may be a kind of a storage facility for intestinal flora.[239] Our gut has resident bacteria that help us to do everything from digest our food to feel happiness. When the gut is flushed, from an episode of diarrhea or from a course of antibiotics, the appendix may help to re-colonize the gut with crucial indigenous bacteria. In fact, *Science* magazine recently reported that scientists today believe that not only is the appendix not a vestige of evolution, but that it has evolved more than 30 times!

The origination of the appendix-as-vestigial theory was actually believed to be Charles Darwin himself. From *Science*:

Charles Darwin was one of the first scientists to theorize on the function of the appendix, which in his day had been identified only in humans and other great apes. He hypothesized that the distant ancestors of these animals survived on a diet of leaves, and so they required a large cecum, a portion of the gut that houses bacteria that can break down stubborn plant tissue. Later, he speculated, these ancestors shifted to a largely fruit-based diet that was easier to digest. A large cecum was no longer necessary, and it began to shrink; today our cecum is tiny. Darwin thought the appendix, which juts off of the cecum, is one of its former folds that shriveled up as the cecum shrank. Consequently, he thought it carried no function.

But some scientists have challenged the idea that the appendix serves no purpose. It's been clear for about a century that the structure contains a particular type of tissue belonging to the lymphatic system. This system carries the white blood cells that help fight infections. Within the last decade, research has shown that this lymphatic tissue encourages the growth of some kinds of beneficial gut bacteria. What's more, careful anatomical study of other mammals has revealed that species as diverse as beavers, koalas, and porcupines also have a structure jutting off of their guts in exactly the same place as our appendix—in other words, the feature is much more common among mammals than once thought. [240]

If you can keep your appendix, you may want to.

Another body part that has had the surgeon's bulls-eye on it intermittently is the prepuce, or foreskin.

In my generation, virtually every male child born was subjected to surgery within the first moments of life. The circumcision rate reached nearly 90% of males born from 1959 through 1971 in the United States.[241] Circumcision was such an ordinary event that the idea of opting out never even touched the consciousness of most American parents before near the turn of the 21st century.

Gerard Tilles of the French Society for the History of Dermatology, writes in the French medical journal *Progres en Urologie*:

> *"Routine circumcision was introduced to the United States in stages beginning in the 1870s for one basic purpose: to deprive the male of a prepuce considered essential for masturbation, a practice thought to be the cause of multiple physical and mental pathologies. From Europe, where masturbation was seen as an indication for circumcision, the fear of masturbation spread to North America, where emphasis was placed on its psychological effects."*

Tilles goes on to describe the bizarre and little-known backstory of circumcision in the U.S. As a routine procedure, it was introduced by then-AMA president Dr. Lewis Sayre, who attributed the existence of the prepuce with a staggering number of "diseases," such as tendon pathology, homosexuality (which was included in the DSM until 1973), alcoholism, epilepsy, asthma, enuresis, kidney disease, gout, prolapse of the rectum, hernia, cancer, syphilis, and, essentially, any unfamiliar or incurable pathology that was encountered. The foreskin was literally treated as a risk factor for men, which is Pathologization in its purest form. By 1929, an editorial in J.A.M.A. called for the circumcision of all newborns, with or without the consent of parents.[242]

"Circumcision became progressively established as a simple health precaution, a kind of surgical vaccination..."

Tilles then describes the process by which routine circumcision began to be scrutinized by a method clearly novel to many doctors of the time: scientific evidence.

"In 1969, Bolande compared circumcision to tonsillectomy, describing both as ritualistic surgeries having no sound scientific basis. He demanded credible scientific evidence showing that circumcision was useful. In the absence of such evidence, he considered circumcision contrary to the most basic principles of medical ethics, principles also highlighted by Price."

In fact, the prepuce is a highly sophisticated structure with a variety of protective functions..
  In "Immunological Functions of the Human Prepuce," P M Fleiss, F M Hodges, and R S Van Howe write:

"A review of the scientific literature, however, reveals that the actual effect of circumcision is the destruction of the clinically-demonstrated hygienic and immunological properties of the prepuce and intact penis."

The article goes on to describe the innate value of this natural body part, as it blocks contaminants from reaching the penis, produces emollients which protect and lubricate the local tissues and enhance the physiology of sexual arousal and intercourse, and contains glands which produce antibacterial substances.

"Today, the most common reason given is that it inhibits the transmission of STDs, even though rigorously controlled studies have consistently shown that circumcised males are at greater risk for all major STDs than males whose penises are intact..."[243]

Today, no national or international medical or scientific community endorses routine circumcision, a surgical procedure once imposed upon infants with neither the parent's consent nor often their knowledge.

Risks engendered by the procedure, include:

- Excessive bleeding
- Infection
- Complications from anesthetics
- Surgical mistakes, including loss of glans and loss of entire penis
- Death (1 in 15,000)
- Extensive scarring
- Skin tags and skin bridges
- Tearing and bleeding at the scar
- Curvature of the penis
- Tight, painful erections
- Difficulty ejaculating
- Impotence

These risks clearly outweigh any medical benefits, which is presumably why the rate of circumcision has been going down consistently over the last several decades and today is hovering around 50%.[244]

Recently, the AAP amended their stance on routine circumcision to include the caveat that circumcision *may* help protect heterosexual men against HIV, but the evidence as it concerns American men is considered only "fair" and the AAP still does not recommend routine circumcision.

Furthermore, if protection against a sexually transmitted disease is the primary benefit to the procedure, then there is no justification for performing it in infancy. At the very least, waiting until the individual is in adolescence affords a measure of informed consent to the patient, whereas the current practice amounts to nonconsensual neonatal cosmetic surgery. Finally, it is interesting to note that female circumcision, which in some cases involves the removal of far less tissue than its male counterpart, has been officially renamed Female Genital Mutilation (FGM), and is considered a human rights violation by the World Health Organization:

"FGM is recognized internationally as a violation of the human rights of girls and women. It reflects deep-rooted inequality between the sexes, and constitutes an extreme form of

*discrimination against women. It is nearly always carried out on minors and is a viola-
tion of the rights of children. The practice also violates a person's rights to health, security
and physical integrity, the right to be free from torture and cruel, inhuman or degrading
treatment, and the right to life when the procedure results in death."*[245]

And so while science is undoubtedly the friend of De-Pathologization, the application
of science is still largely in the hands of the Pathologizers. This means that substantive
change is likely to come, as it did in the case of circumcision, from a grass-roots shift
in consciousness. Circumcision rates were driven down initially by parents who dared
to challenge the status quo of ritualistic medicine, often against the gradient of their
doctors' recommendations. Course-corrections of this nature often require action on
the part of those outside the cultural core who operate (literally) in the momentum
of mainstream thinking. It is in this endeavor that this book operates.

Honestly, we only need to be confronted with one instance of modern medical procedures being perpetuated long after the evidence should have banished the practice
in order to now have the onus on us, the public, to question any practice, ritual, treatment or therapy that is part of the culture of medicine. This is our responsibility no
matter how deeply engrained the practice is in our culture or how much hostility
or coercion we may encounter in that resistance. In fact, I would suggest that the
greater the emotional energy around the response to questioning a treatment, the
more imperative it may be to question it.

CHAPTER 20
Born to Run

Even an act as simple and elemental as running has not been immune to pathological reframing. In his book, *Born To Run*,[246] journalist and former war correspondent Christopher MacDougall describes the fascinating history of the modern running shoe and the unspoken truth of its flaws.

The story begins as MacDougall, a runner, consults his doctor about a running injury, the latest in a long series of running injuries. His doctor tells him that the cause of the injury is running itself.

"Running is your problem," Dr. Joe Torg told him.

"But I'm barely running at all," said MacDougall.

"The human body is not designed for that kind of abuse...," said Dr. Torg.

Torg, as MacDougall would point out, should know. He helped create the entire field of sports medicine and is the co-author of *The Running Athlete*, the definitive textbook on running injuries.

"Up to eight out of ten runners are hurt every year. It doesn't matter if you're heavy or thin, speedy or slow, a marathon champ or a weekend huffer, you're just as likely to savage your knees, shins, hamstrings, hips, or heels...No invention yet has slowed the carnage; you can now buy running shoes with steel bedsprings embedded in the soles and Adidas that adjust their cushioning by microchip, but the injury rate hasn't decreased a jot in thirty years. If anything it's actually ebbed up; Achilles tendon blowouts have seen a ten percent increase."

The explanation that the medical world gives should by now be predictable:

Running is inherently pathological.

"Just as repeated hammering on an apparently impenetrable rock will eventually reduce the stone to dust, the impact loads associated with running can ultimately break down your bones, cartilage, muscles, tendons, and ligaments," claims the *Sports Injury Bulletin.*

A report by the American Association of Orthopedic Surgeons concluded that distance running is "an outrageous threat to the integrity of the knee."

That comment about the hammering of the force of running on the soft tissues of the body caught my eye. Then I remembered where I had heard it: Joseph DeLee, the father of modern obstetrics, described the forces of labor as "repetitive pounding of the baby's head against the perineum." The image he invoked was one of a soft, delicate fetal cranium being crushed by the concrete-like perineum. He even attributed this "pounding" as a cause of brain damage. In reality, the perineum is soft, not hard, and the baby's head is remarkably pliant, flexible, and durable. It is composed of loosely arranged cartilage plates that can bend, flex, and absorb a tremendous amount of force. The fact is that both the perineum and the baby's head were designed, through the ruthless process of evolution, to "withstand" the forces of labor. Our very existence is evidence of it.

Similarly, the pronouncement that running is inherently "bad" for humans is based not on science, but on experience. The danger of this practice is that we extrapolate limited data to make larger statements about fundamental capacities.

"Know what I'd recommend?" Dr. Torg concluded as he prepared to deliver an injection of cortisone to the author's foot, "Buy a bike."

So MacDougall went for a second opinion, another shot, and a recommendation to quit running. And a third opinion, all of which he summed up as:

"How come my foot hurts?
Because running is bad for you.
Why is running bad for me?
Because it makes your foot hurt.

Then MacDougall discovered the Tarahumara, a group of Mexican Indians living in the Copper Canyons. To say that the Tarahumara were avid runners would be like saying that Michael Jordan could bounce a ball. Tarahumara runners regularly travel over a hundred miles a day through the treacherous steep canyon trails that surround them. One runner once ran 435 miles, and others have been reported to run for 300 miles at a time. That's nearly 12 full marathons. The regular running parties the Tarahumara throw include an all-night party that concludes in the morning with a *two* day long running race that covers over a hundred miles.

All in flimsy, thin-soled Huarache sandals.

MacDougall asks the obvious question:

"How come they're not crippled? It's as if a clerical error entered the stats in the wrong columns: Shouldn't we, the ones with state-of-the-art running shoes and custom-made esthetics, have the zero casualty rate, and the Tarahumara, who run way more, on way rockier terrain, in shoes that barely qualify as shoes, be constantly banged up? Their legs are just tougher, since they've been running all their lives, I thought, before catching my own goof. But that means they should be hurt more, not less. If running is bad for your legs, then running lots should be a lot worse."

The answer to that question was staggering: The very shoes that were designed to give us the competitive edge and protect us from injuries were actually causing them.

The modern running shoe was designed by Bill Bowerman, whose company eventually became Nike. Before the first Nike, runners through the ages had virtually identical form: back straight, feet moving in a "stroking" motion, the foot strike occurring under the center of gravity, the force being distributed from the outer edge of the mid-foot, across the foot, then off the toes. Running shoes were thin-soled, had no arch support or ankle pronation control, and little to no cushioning. The cover of Jim Fixx's *Complete Book of Running* show his famous muscular legs in mid-stride wearing what amounts to a thin wafer of plastic under a simple nylon upper.

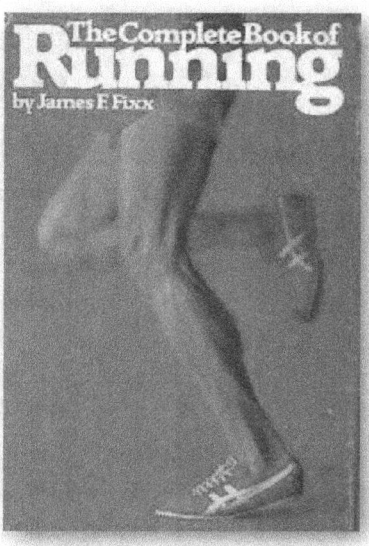

The first Nike running shoe, the Cortez, operated on the unprecedented (and untested) premise that by altering the natural running stride of the human being, one could lengthen the stride and increase overall speed. This involved incorporating a running form no human had ever employed, in which the lead leg is thrown forward, ahead of the center of gravity, and instead of landing bent and absorbing the force, the leg is straight and the force is transmitted directly into the knee, hip and spine. Of course, the idea was to insert cushioning into the shoe to diminish that force. Unfortunately, it would not be until nearly 40 years later that that theory would actually be tested.

Dr. Daniel Lieberman, professor of biological anthropology at Harvard University, states,

"A lot of foot and knee injuries that are currently plaguing us are actually caused by people running with shoes that actually make our feet weak, cause us to over-pronate, give us knee problems. Until 1972, when the modern athletic shoe was invented by Nike, people ran in very thin-soled shoes, had strong feet, and had much lower incidence of knee injuries."

Lieberman has recently published follow-up studies which support his findings.

MacDougall tells the story of Coach Vin Lananna of the Stanford University track and cross-country teams, who trained his runners barefoot because he found they ran faster with less injuries. His results? "In just ten years at Stanford, Lananna's track and cross-country teams had won five NCAA team championships and twenty-two individual titles, and Lananna himself had been named NCAA Cross-Country Coach of the Year. Lananna had already sent three runners to the Olympics..."

The modern running shoe fails to prevent injuries because it inhibits the natural mechanisms of injury prevention. When you place your foot in a shoe, those mechanisms turn off. That's why modern barefoot runners call them "coffins for the foot." The padding insulates the sensors of the foot from feeling the ground. The technology of the shoe is designed to replace the innate protective mechanisms, so those mechanisms turn off.

"Putting your feet in shoes is similar to putting them in a plaster cast," says Dr. Hartmann. "If I put your leg in plaster, we'll find forty to sixty percent atrophy of the musculature within six weeks. Something similar happens to your feet when they're encased in shoes."

MacDougall continues:

But instead of doctors leading the charge for a muscular foot, it was turning into a class war pitting podiatrists against their own patients. Barefoot advocates like Drs. Brand and Hartmann were still rare, while traditional podiatric thinking still saw human feet as Nature's Mistake, a work in progress that could always be improved by a little scalpel-sculpting and orthotic reshaping...That "born broken" mentality found its perfect expression in The Runners' Repair Manual. *Written by Dr. Murray Weisenfeld, a leading sports podiatrist...[it] begins with this dire pronouncement:*

"Man's foot was not originally designed for walking, much less running long distances."

Take a moment to consider the audacity of that statement. Man, the product of millions of years of evolution, whose name, *homo erectus*, literally means "upright man," is being described as somehow lacking the capacity to tolerate his own adaptation of being upright. This kind of nonsense is simply incompatible with evolutionary theory. It is akin to claiming that flying is bad for birds or fish are poorly adapted for life in water. It is a paradigm that our acceptance of Pathologization enables: If our bodies are incapable of something as elemental as birthing, why would we not be similarly misshapen when it comes to ambulation?

The modern "scientific" story that running is inherently bad/dangerous/damaging to humans is further refuted by the evidence of long distance running in humans as an integral part of our hunter/gatherer existence. The Tarahumara are not the only tribe who run for long distances. "Persistence hunting" is now believed to have been an integral part of human evolution. This is hunting by perseverance: literally running down prey.

Your initial reaction is probably, yeah, right, a human chasing down a deer? How is *that* possible? Well, it is not only possible, it is likely the only thing that kept our great-great-great-great (etc.) grandparents alive for about 40,000 years, before the development of the spear, atl-atl, and other long distance hunting tools. Humans have evolved special adaptations peculiar to long distance running that make us not just *good* distance runners, but *the best*.

One key is sweat. In order to keep up the metabolic rate necessary for sustained running, mammals need to sweat or pant. However, prey animals like deer and gazelle are covered in fur; they can't sweat very well. As a result, their endurance is limited. In fact, once an animal's body temperature reaches 105 degrees, it will simply stop. Humans have lost nearly all their fur; we can sweat extremely well. And as long as we sweat, we can run, providing we have a water source to replenish our bodies.

Most mammals can only take one breath per stride. This limits their endurance. Humans are the only mammals in existence that can take more, and we do, double to triple that of our prey. Being upright also limits the amount of direct sun exposure, thereby limiting heat buildup. That's why we still have lots of hair on our heads; it is the area of greatest solar heat contact; the hair insulates our brains (our brains also have special adaptation in the form of a unique venous cooling system that help keep it air-conditioned during prolonged exposure).

The end result is a creature that is the greatest long distance runner on the planet. We can run down ANYTHING. Antelopes, deer, gazelle, you name it. These animals generally will sprint away from a predator then stop. But a deer's sprinting speed is only a little faster than a human's long distance jogging speed. Before long, the human catches up. As long as we can track the same animal, it will eventually overheat and simply lay down. Native Americans would actually walk right up to the deer and smother it with their hands! These kills were considered sacred because the animal's hide was not punctured in any way.

How about horses? Does this mean a human could outrun a horse? Could, has, and continues to. The 50-mile Man Against Horse Race in Prescott, Arizona is won by a human just about every year (Horses come closer to humans because they have an unusually well-developed capacity to sweat. These horses are, however, given plentiful water and high energy food to sustain them in the competition. A prey animal would not have this luxury).

I was one of the millions of runners captivated by MacDougall's argument. Like many runners, I had been plagued by injuries, despite investing in the most expensive running shoes and adapting my running in every conceivable way. I had plantar fasciitis, sore ankles, knee, hip, and back problems, and Achilles tendonitis. My last pair of running shoes cost $150.

I acquired a pair of Vibram Five Fingers and began to run in them. I vividly recall stepping onto the trail with these flimsy slippers on my feet and feeling an uneasiness bordering on fear. I felt as if I was stepping into a battle with nothing but a cardboard shield and a Nerf sword. It was a leap of faith. Immediately, though, my body reverted into a new (old), natural, abbreviated, comfortable, fast style and rhythm of running that I had utilized any time I had run barefoot, over lawns, in the sand at the beach, or even across the hardwood floors of my house.

Within a few weeks I was putting in the same mileage as I had in my super-high tech Salomons. The only difference was that now the painful ankle problem I had been experiencing was mysteriously gone. So was the sore knee and hip, and the creeping plantar fasciitis. In fact, I hadn't felt this good running in years, despite the fact that I had eliminated all cushioning, arch support, tread, heel stabilizers, and pronation control. My body was providing all of those things. As I ran I could feel my arches flexing and springing as my foot absorbed the force of the stride and rebounded that force back into the push-off. My stride naturally shortened so my feet were underneath me. I no longer rolled my ankles or overextended my Achilles tendon with unnaturally long strides. I was stable, balanced, bouncy, and light, all courtesy of my own body, not technology.

It has now been seven years. My arches have not collapsed, my knees have not crumpled. In fact, my joints and arches are feeling healthier and lighter than ever before.

With the obvious caveat for scale, how different was this experience than that of the modern woman giving birth at home without the massive technologies of the hospital? Technologies which promised to enhance performance but in reality shut off critical natural innate mechanisms, our own evolutionary technologies, the products not of decades of research but of millennia of trial and error in the real world. Modern running shoes are described as "coffins" because the artificial technology of the shoe inhibits the natural technology of your foot. In the same way, the modern hospital birth inhibits the natural technology of the birthing woman's body by removing the critical environmental conditions upon which those mechanisms depend. It's like removing a trigger from a gun and trying to fire it, then designating all guns as faulty.

The point here is not to dispose of all modern technology as useless and sopho-moric. Clearly, medicine and technology have value. The examples here describe, how-ever, the complementary extremist position: to dismiss the human body and its inherent capacities as universally incompetent and inferior to modern science. Redefining nor-mal, natural body processes as inherently pathological is not only arbitrary but extrem-ist. Clear and definite limitations exist in the scientific model. It operates poorly in open systems; accommodates poorly for intangibles such as emotion, belief, and relation-ships; and is easily corrupted by the capitalistic model, since the net product of sci-ence is very often an actual product which is then marketed and sold by companies or corporations. Hence, we should always exercise a healthy skepticism about scientific proclamations, particularly when they involve "science" telling us that we are intrinsi-cally incompetent, and thus require (usually expensive) technological assistance.

An ideal system of thought is one which begins with not only an acknowledgement of the inherent capacities of the human body, but, perhaps even more importantly, an acknowledgement that at this point we clearly do not fully know or appreciate the full scale of those capacities. We must, in other words, not only acknowledge what we know the body can do, but also that which we don't yet know the body can do.

Slipping my feet into a pair of rubber slippers and taking off for a run was a leap of faith. Everything modern science had taught me told me that my body was inherently incapable of performing this action without damaging myself. That an act as elemen-tal and intrinsically human as simply running barefoot can be so effectively reframed that even I, a person who has learned to trust the body in the face of extreme medical reframing, would have such a deeply ingrained belief system about my own body and its capacities, speaks to the insidious way in which this reframing takes place.

CHAPTER 21

Pathologization of a Star

n December of 2009, cancer groups, like the RayFesta melanoma foundation, blasted comedian Rosie O'Donnell for comments she made about...the sun. News of the controversy made national headlines. The cancer group called O'Donnell's comments "irresponsible" and "misinformed." What was the quote that got her into trouble?

This one:

"I live to tan...exposure to the sun isn't dangerous...."

On the surface, it may be difficult to understand the controversy. Exposure to the sun is not only not intrinsically dangerous, it is essential to life. Many early cultures worshipped the sun for good reason. It is the source of all life on our planet. Exposure to the sun allows humans to manufacture Vitamin D naturally. Vitamin D is essential to human health. Without it, our bones bend and fold and deform. In children, that's called rickets. In the U.S., rickets was a major health catastrophe. What was one of the causes of the rickets epidemic? Lack of sun exposure.

Furthermore, while there is statistically a link between certain kinds of sun exposure and the incidence of melanoma in certain individuals, the specifics are actually in Ms. O'Donnell's favor. An overview of scientific studies published in the *International Journal of Cancer*[247] found that cancer risks were elevated in people who were *sunburned* either in childhood or adulthood. Interestingly, cancer risk was also elevated in individuals who experienced "intermittent exposure." What was the one group mentioned who had "significantly reduced risk?" Those with "heavy occupational exposure." In other words, people with tans.

On a deeper level, the outrage that these melanoma groups expressed at O'Donnell's comments is a powerful reflection of the degree to which the process of "Pathologization" has developed in the psyche of so many Americans.

Childbirth used to be a normal, natural event. In the hands of medicine, it has been reduced to the excision of a tumor. In an interesting bit of history, it turns out that one of the primary causes of birth complications in the 17th century, which partially enabled the universal medicalization of birth in the U.S. was deformed pelvises from lack of sun exposure.

In the case of melanoma, we have Pathologization put to the extreme. When faced with the rising incidence of melanoma and few real answers from a system that has only drugs, radiation, and surgery as its solutions, we are left with one option:

Blame the sun.

We have to ask how different this is from the medieval physicians blaming illness and disease on the movement of the planets and stars. Childbed fever, the scourge of Europe in the 1800s, was believed to be caused by astrological or meteorological phenomena.

We can only hope that the process of Pathologization will become so extreme and conspicuous that a revolt against the extremism of the medical paradigm will erupt and a more balanced approach to health will emerge, one in which the very real and irreplaceable gifts of modern medicine are designated to those arenas in which they serve the public best—emergency, life-saving care—while the larger task of promoting and maintaining health is mediated by a diverse body of professionals, which may include medicine, but is not governed by the medical paradigm. What paradigm is appropriate for the task of health promotion? One which is based on the idea that health comes from within, and often so does illness, and one that sees that the solutions to many health problems lie in enhancing the health of the individual rather than finding an exterior cause to implicate and attack, such as a bacteria, a virus, a gene...or a *star*.

CHAPTER 22
Evidence-Based Medicine

As I've mentioned a few times over the course of this book, one of the most common questions I get in my lectures and classes is, "How are unproven or unsafe procedures perpetuated in health care beyond the point where we know they don't work, or, we know we *don't know whether they do* work?"

When you go to your doctor, you are presuming that the treatments you are receiving have been vetted through a scientific process and have shown reliability in helping your condition. In fact, a central element of the discussion in which this book is engaged is, what are the risks associated with displacing our trust in our bodies and placing it in the hands of the specialty fields of medicine and pharmacology? Much of the work that I encounter in my chiropractic practice is with patients who are struggling to reconcile the blind faith they are encouraged to have in western medicine (and its consistent suggestion that alternative methods and philosophies are illegitimate) with the vague awareness of a far greater degree of fallibility and limited vision than they are being led to believe exists.

Evidence-based medicine is a great idea conceptually, promoting the utilization of tools that have been proven to be effective. EBM is medicine's response to its own history of promoting and utilizing tools that were never subjected to the scrutiny of science, never tested, yet in many cases these methods were defended to the point of a kind of rabid dogmatism. The perpetuation of unproven or disproven procedures, from bloodletting and purging to episiotomies and C-sections, is a legacy that is as much a part of the history of Western medicine as any other clinical strategy.

History is replete with medical misinformation...

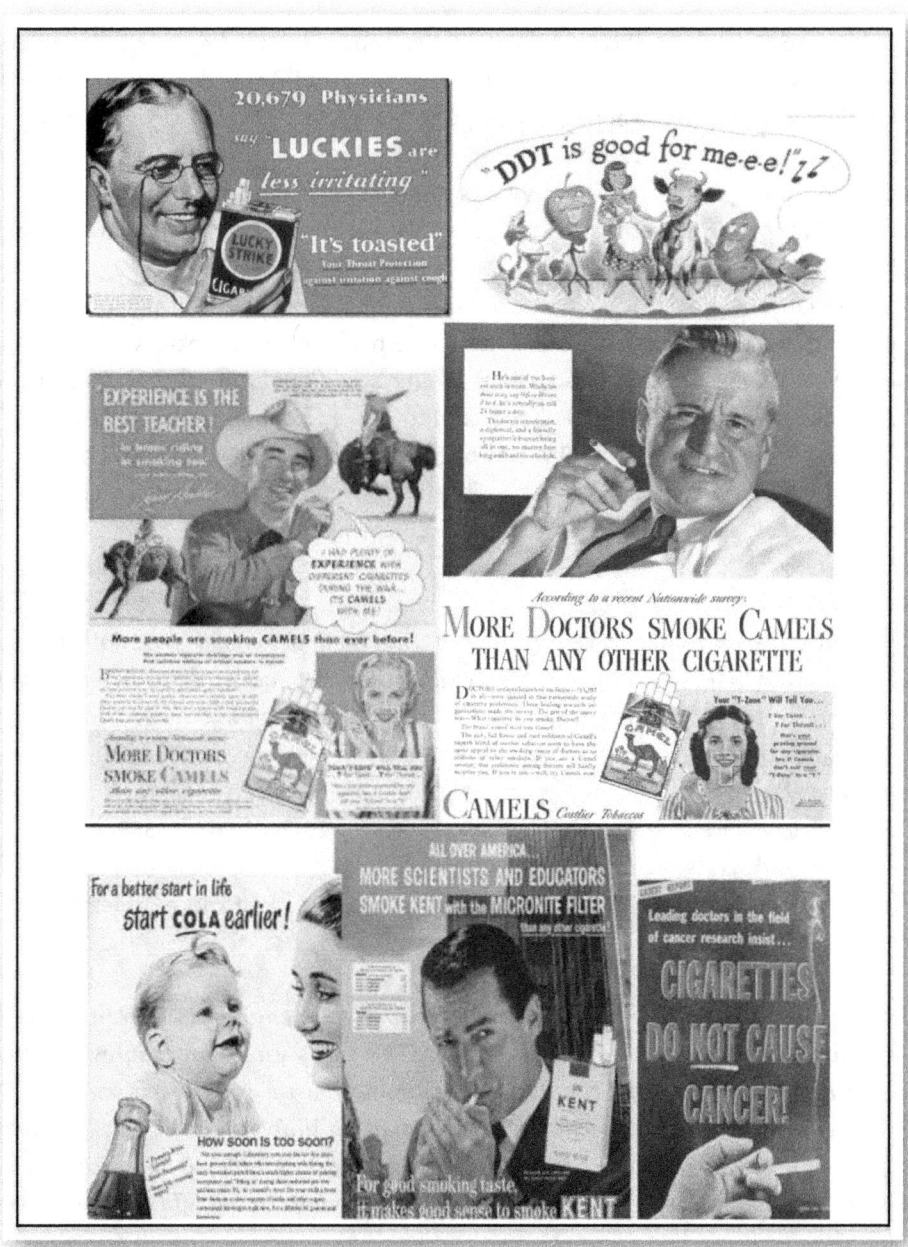

But the general impression we are taught to have about medicine is that, by and large, it is evolving scientifically and disposing of unproven methods in favor of proven ones. As Starr and others have noted, up to the early 20th century, medicine was largely based on ritual and theory and unburdened by evidence. Bloodletting, hanging, leeches, purging, and the use of highly toxic substances like mercury were the tools of a trade which had not yet integrated the ethics of science into its procedures. Surgery was perhaps an exception in this sense, since the survival of the patient provided immediate and irrevocable clinical feedback on efficacy.

The current movement to articulate EBM with modern medical procedures is migrating into the discussion around alternative health care methods. A kind of sanctimony has permeated these discussions, as any lack of randomized clinical testing of alternative methods is being used as a tool to discredit those methods, despite the fact that the very concept of EBM was only introduced in 1992,[248] at which point it was labeled "a new approach," and it has been poorly integrated into medical practice itself. Sacket, et al., in CMAJ, exemplifies this embarrassingly:

"Without evidence from positive randomized trials (and, better still, systematic reviews of randomized trials), we cannot justify soliciting the well to accept any personal health intervention...to satisfy a narcissistic need for public acclaim or in a misguided attempt to do good, advocate 'preventive' maneuvers that have never been validated in rigorous randomized trials."

-The Arrogance of Preventive Medicine, CMAJ Aug 20, 2002 167 (4) 363-4

However, the integration of science with medicine has been more imperfect than people might think.

"For much of the century the medical profession assumed that its scientific knowledge about the body and about disease had driven its use of procedures. Patients also generally accepted the procedures, assuming that they had been scientifically validated. But for many procedures, this assumption simply was not true. The deputy director of the Rockefeller Foundation estimated that only 10-20 percent of all clinical interventions used in 1980 were based on demonstrated efficacy and safety. Although medicine had competed with other healing professions on the grounds that it alone was scientific, it had neglected to apply the scientific method to evaluating its own work."

-Barbara Bridgman Perkins, *Medical Delivery Business*

Perkins notes Ernest Amory Codman, who advocated for the "radical proposal" that hospitals actually keep track of whether patients lived or died after being released. His reward was to be "excoriated by his colleagues" and forced to leave his position at Mass Gen. Hospital. Unlike Semmelveiss, he was ultimately vilified by the emergence of EBM in the 1990s, but as Perkins acutely points out:

"The remarkable and rather appalling implication of the popularity of EBM at that time was the extent to which medicine throughout the century had not been evidence-based.

"After Codman, accusations of excessive procedures and unnecessary surgery rumbled within the profession, albeit at a low level. By the last third of the century, it was accepted in some medical as well as planning and payer circles that the use of many medical procedures vastly exceeded scientific evidence of their benefit."

Califano charged in 1988 that at least 60% and perhaps as many as 80% of all coronary artery bypass graft operations, more than 50% of cardiac pacemaker implants, and at least 50% of Cesarean sections performed in the U.S. were unnecessary.

In the field of obstetrics, according to Perkins, "The first systematic medical approach to assessing perinatal efficacy was obstetrician Ian Chalmers's work in Britain's National Perinatal Epidemiology Unit [1989]. The unit's studies and research analyses empirically demonstrated the inadequacy of evidentiary support for many routine perinatal practices."

In 1978, the U.S. Office of Technology Assessment (OTA) reported: "Only 10%-20% of all procedures currently used in medical practice have been shown to be efficacious by controlled trial." (83) In 1995, the OTA compared medical technology in eight countries (Australia, Canada, France, Germany, the Netherlands, Sweden, the UK, and the U.S.) and again noted that few medical procedures in the U.S. have been subjected to clinical trial.

The fact that, increasingly, the primary imperative of medical doctors, and in particular obstetricians, is becoming self-protection from lawsuit engenders an ecosystem in which procedures and protocols are fueled by safety to the doctor rather than to the patient. Evidence-based medicine is an ethic which at times competes directly with the malpractice risk of the doctor. This is an inhospitable environment for the former. Proof of this fact can be found in the long list of currently accepted procedures which remain part of the standard medical protocol not only in the absence of evidence, but against the gradient of evidence (see chapter 9).

Data from current medical practices, subjected to the scrutiny of evidence, shows a surprising lack of scientific validation. A recent study published by the *British Medical Journal*[249] showed the results of an analysis of 2,500 common medical treatments and found the following:

- 13 percent were found to be beneficial.
- 23 percent were likely to be beneficial.
- Eight percent were as likely to be harmful as beneficial.
- Six percent were unlikely to be beneficial.
- Four percent were likely to be harmful or ineffective.

This means that when you take your sick child to the doctor, there is only a 36 percent chance that he will receive treatment that has been scientifically proven to be either beneficial or even likely to be beneficial. A recent meta-review of conventional medical practices concluded that eight percent of treatments were positive and 62 percent were negative or showed "no evidence of effect."[250]

John P.A. Ioannidis, chief of the Prevention Research Center at Stanford University, and medicine's top "myth-buster," has set out to subject biomedical research to its own standards of proof: evidence and data.

His question: How many biomedical studies are wrong?

His answer is shocking: most.

"'People are being hurt and even dying" because of false medical claims, he says, "not quackery, but errors in medical research," reports Sharon Begley in *Newsweek*.[251] Ioannidis' early work debunked several claims that certain genes were the cause of illnesses like Parkinson's (debunked in 2010) and cardiovascular disease (2009). Begley writes: "Geneticists have mostly mended their ways, tightening statistical criteria, but other fields still need to clean house," Ioannidis says.

One could go on and on, but I can summarize by simply and confidently stating that if we are to dismiss complementary and alternative medicine purely on the basis of lack of rigorous objective study, then we must also dismiss a substantial number of western medical practices currently in use.

This information should not necessarily deter a person from seeking out medical care for an urgent health concern, but it should impart perhaps a more realistic view of medicine's fallibility, and, more importantly, recognize the limitations of the medical paradigm to accomplish the larger goal of public health and wellness. And when doctors discourage their patients from forgoing medical treatments in favor of alternative approaches, including no treatment whatsoever, on the basis of "unproven" therapies, the patient may want to take that advice with a grain or two of salt.

Furthermore, the standard tools of EBM may not afford the adequate insight into the mechanisms and efficacy of alternative therapies that would be necessary in order to determine their value.

As important as it is for the medical community to understand more fully the efficacy of natural health care, it is even more important for them to understand the distinction between the core paradigms of allopathic and wellness-based care. For the mainstream medical community, still operating under a strict biomedical model, the randomized controlled trial, or RCT, is the gold standard because it represents the epitome of reductionist thinking.

In this model, factors such as faith/belief, relationships, expectations, emotional and psychological states, and spiritual perspectives are intangibles which, since they cannot be currently quantified, must be wholly disregarded. While this is a clinical necessity for the purposes of research protocol congruity, it is nevertheless arguable as to whether it accurately represents the actual nature of the dynamic interactions occurring in the health care environment, particularly the holistic health care environment, in which these factors are not only accepted as valid, but actually integrated into a strategy for care. In other words, it may be a valid system for researchers, but not for patients or practitioners.

The bio-psychosocial model, credited to Engel in 1972[252] but in reality an extension of many eastern health philosophies, which have been intact for thousands of years, is representative of many complementary and alternative medicine (CAM) practices. In this model, the patient's relationships—to the practitioner, to him or herself, to the patient's family, friends, co-workers—all represent not barriers to research efficacy, but critical elements of it.

In these models, RCT is not only not the "gold standard"; it is, on a practical level, a limited approach which fails to accommodate many important elements of the healing relationship. The unique challenges to RCT methodology cited by researchers are, in many cases, perfectly valid and important components of the healing dynamic for the holistic practitioner, such as "relationship with the practitioner." RCT is a poor study framework in these cases because it neglects to integrate the treatment protocol into its own paradigm. The paradigm of holistic health is that belief, relationships, emotions, expectations OF COURSE influence the outcome. They are not obstacles to the pursuit of truth; they are essential ground rules for the pursuit of truth.

As Smith and Bell pithily noted in their *British Medical Journal* paper entitled, "Parachute use to prevent death and major trauma related to gravitational challenge: systematic review of randomised controlled trials":

> *"As with many interventions intended to prevent ill health, the effectiveness of parachutes has not been subjected to rigorous evaluation by using randomised controlled trials. Advocates of evidence based medicine have criticised the adoption of interventions evaluated by using only observational data. We think that everyone might benefit if the most radical protagonists of evidence based medicine organised and participated in a double blind, randomised, placebo controlled, crossover trial of the parachute..."[253]*

The medical community not only needs to understand the world of CAM better, it needs to understand the fundamental paradigm of CAM, and consider whether incompatibilities in paradigms and research models are a formula for flawed research data. Subjecting holistic health care to allopathic systems of validation may influence the potential for the care to be fairly assessed.

Rather than asking, "How can we get more RCT studies done on alternative care?" perhaps a better question may be, "Is a western allopathic model of research optimal for a system of treatment with which it has core fundamental incompatibilities?" The question is not whether there should be a burden of proof upon any health care practice or technique, but rather whether there can be one single model for proof that can be universally applied to a complex and broad range of methods and clinical objectives.

We must also be concerned with the potential for corruption in the advancement of EBM. Ioannidis' research pointed to funding bias as a common source of research manipulation: When the manufacturer of the drug pays for the studies of its safety and effectiveness, it has a conflict of interest in publishing damning results. The skewing is not in the methodology, but rather in the simple selection of which studies get published.

The *New England Journal of Medicine* published a recent article called, "Dangerous Deception — Hiding the Evidence of Adverse Drug Effects."[254]

"The health care system has a hard time performing drug-safety analyses, in large part because it relies on the pharmaceutical industry to conduct most research on the risks and benefits of medications. It is naive to expect companies to voluntarily fund studies that could sink lucrative products, the FDA lacks the regulatory clout to require them, and despite the $220 billion we spend on drugs each year, we apparently can't find the resources to provide public support for these studies, even if the results could be of great clinical importance and save millions of dollars."

Therefore, while the RCT is a valid and valuable tool for investigating scientific hypotheses, its limitations must be acknowledged, particularly with respect to applications in fields, which operate under new and advancing paradigms.

And while randomized controlled studies remain the gold standard for alternative modality research for the medical community, RESULTS remain the gold standard for the actual patients. Given that Americans spend more money out of pocket for alternative practitioners than for allopathic physicians, it is reasonable to postulate that many of these practices are achieving results that their competition is reluctant to acknowledge. For patients, the only real "evidence" in Evidence-Based Medicine is RESULTS: Will this work for me? One would have to admit that it is quite an insult to the average health care consumer that (s)he would be effectively solicited to pay out of pocket for techniques that do not produce results. In the case of the medical profession, we have a social system of compliance and a universal surrender of private judgment which empowers that kind of decision, but success in the highly competitive alternative field is so intensely dependent upon clinical results that to suggest that such motives as "narcissism" or "misguided altruism" would be sustainable in this market is, to the actual alternative care provider, laughable.

The limitations of EBM are representative of the limitations of medicine itself. EBM and RCTs are the products of a myopically mechanistic, reductionist model of human health and physiology. This is congruent with the constructs of allopathic medicine, and thus EBM works well as a research tool for that purpose.

But utilizing RCTs as the "gold standard" for non-allopathic fields, or for the broader imperatives of well-being, without discriminating their respective paradigms in the mechanistic/vitalistic spectrum, is a recapitulation of the fatal flaws that we have recounted in this book—that of applying a "cookie-cutter," one-size-fits-all strategy to an open system which is anything but one-sized. To a certain degree, it represents the narrowness that has plagued medicine since its rise to prominence in the mid 1800s. And to a certain degree it speaks to the professional agenda of medicine as a social and political structure: to maintain its monopoly on health care by claiming to be the ultimate arbiter of truth and homogenizing the dialogue into exclusively medical terms and measurements.

Research models exist and are being actively developed for holistic health care systems. In the field of chiropractic, Network Spinal Care has adopted a research model, which is congruent with the bio-psychosocial model, and applied it to its own program of evidence-based investigations with a high degree of success. Emerging models of research need to adapt to emerging understandings of health and wellness, many of which extend beyond the biomedical model of allopathic medicine and the RCTs, which can, under ideal conditions, measure its success well.

CHAPTER 23
Trust: De-Pathologizing Your Life

"Edges are important because they define a limitation in order to deliver us from it. When we come to an edge we come to a frontier that tells us that we are now about to become more than we have been before. As long as one operates in the middle of things, one can never really know the nature of the medium in which one moves."
-WILLIAM IRWIN THOMPSON

The story of Pathologization is the story of each of us, of our potentialities and the amazing capacity of our bodies to heal, from within, naturally and powerfully. The foundation of allopathic medicine as the exclusive arbiter of the American health care system has had many positive consequences, particularly in the field of emergency medicine and life-saving medical procedures. It centralized and codified emerging therapeutics and created a licensing framework for maintaining and improving care. A negative consequence of this relationship, however, has been the Pathologization of many of our amazing biological abilities and the establishment of a wide range of technologies which have the tendency to interfere with and disrupt these normal body processes. In the case of a swollen ankle or upset stomach, the disruption may be minor. In the case of our deeply troubled American maternity care system, the disruption is not only massive, but the consequences can be quite literally fatal.

We need a balanced approach to the body in which the value of modern technologies would be considered with respect not only to their intrinsic value, but also to the degree to which they may interfere with or disrupt a natural process. Weighing risks and benefits is a process which should include as much valid information as possible. Opening our minds to larger paradigms reveals a broader range of information upon which we can base these decisions. Dispelling old mythologies about the innate character of the human body is an essential element of this course-correction, on both a global and personal scale.

De-Pathologization is a path you can begin on today.

Our new model endorses the utilization of medicine and technology with restraint and intelligence, to constantly be asking the question: Is this an improvement, or are we mucking things up in a very flashy and expensive way?

One of the key messages of "Trust" is that we must, as health care consumers, as owners of our bodies, constantly question the stories we are told about our own biology. Awareness of the "Handy Hammer" phenomenon empowers us to look more closely at the rituals many of us have embraced or inherited over the years, and question whether they are based in science, or in ritual itself.

A greater understanding of our bodies' capacity to heal and perform highly sophisticated functions opens exciting new directions for choices in how to support and promote that healing capacity. While "preventive" medicine is still pouring its resources into detecting and treating disease in ourselves, our children, our grandchildren, we can choose to devote our own resources into truly preventing illness and disease by addressing the actual environmental factors which consistently cause it, such as diet, exercise, weight control, reduction of toxins in our food, air, water, and living spaces, and a host of "alternative" systems which promote health and wellness rather than avoiding disease.

The effect of De-Pathologizing and embracing Trust, when appropriate, on future generations, can be massive. The expression of health promotion in the Trust paradigm extends beyond how we manage our bodies because, outside of the medical model, we can see that we are a part of our environment, and dependent on it for our survival. Health promotion then becomes as much about environmentalism, social justice, and global perspectives as it is about how we manage our own personal health. In our chiropractic office, our outcome assessment protocol includes tracking the degree to which enhanced sense of connection within the patient is promoting any changes in the patient's relationship to their spheres of social interrelationships, from interpersonal to global.

Here is an example of a typical patient response:

7) Using a scale of 1 to 5, where 1 is the least and 5 is the most, please evaluate your experience of the following, both before starting care, and now:

	Before	Now
Trust your inner instincts, or inner voice	1 ②3 4 5	1 2③4 5
Feel connected to others at work	1 ②3 4 5	1 2③4 5
Feel connected to others at play	1 ②3 4 5	1 2③4 5
Feel whole	1 ②3 4 5	1 2③4 5
Disturbed by sudden life changes	1 2 3 ④5	1②3 4 5
Disturbed by predictability or sameness	1 ②3 4 5	1②3 4 5
Restfulness of sleep	1 2③4 5	1 2③4 5
Eager to take on new projects	1 ②3 4 5	1 2 3④5
Hold on to tensions, anxiety	1 ②③④5	1②3 4 5
Hold a grudge	1 2 3④5	1②3 4 5
Feel compassion towards others	1 2③4 5	1 2 3④5
Feel responsible towards your environment	1 ②③4 5	1 2③4 5
Feel symptoms and observe them	1②3 4 5	1 2 3④5
Feel symptoms with getting disturbed or frightened	1 2③4 5	1②3 4 5
Bounce back from physical trauma	1 2③4 5	1 2③4 5
Bounce back from emotional trauma	1 2③4 5	1 2 3④5
Bounce back from mental stress	1 2③4 5	1 2 3④5
Bounce back from sickness, or symptom episodes	1②3 4 5	1 2 3④5
Aware of what my body wants from me	1②3 4 5	1 2③④5
Aware of what I need to eat	1②3 4 5	1 2 3④5
Aware of what does not work for me	1②3 4 5	1 2 3④5
Express my needs to others	1②3 4 5	1 2③4 5
Take responsibility for areas of my life	1②3 4 5	1 2 3④5
Unwind from my tensions	1②3 4 5	1 2③4 5
Spontaneously express emotions	1②3 4 5	1 2③4 5
Feel empowered in life	1②3 4 5	1 2③4 5
Experience peace	1②3 4 5	1 2③4 5
Experience greater self-awareness	1②3 4 5	1 2 3④5
Ability to spontaneously forgive myself	1②3 4 5	1 2③4 5
Ability to spontaneously forgive others	1②3 4 5	1 2③4 5
Ability to self heal	1②3 4 5	1 2③4 5

Performing these holistic evaluations of patient well-being as an evolving dynamic opened our eyes to the dramatic impact of wellness-based chiropractic. Our patients were not just experiencing more ease and happiness in their bodies, they were experiencing consistent improvements in their quality of life in a dramatically complex arena of elemental life relationships. This evaluation demonstrated a noticeable improvement in the patient's quality of life in areas such as personal empowerment, emotional resilience, empathy and compassion, and interpersonal communication—even though none of our therapies were directed at those elements of her wellness. Out of 31 parameters studied, a typical patient like this experienced improvement in 18 parameters and significant improvement in 10 parameters, and reported no change in only 3.

Applying a model of care which recognizes, embraces, and integrates the diversity of factors impacting well-being creates an environment for those factors to integrate into the patient experience in a positive way.

Furthermore, simply utilizing these evaluations also affirmed to our patients that we understood that their well-being was about more than their back or neck pain.

This in turn affirmed that the unfolding quality of their life involved a process in which they were clearly participants, not just observers.

Integrating, or re-integrating the very important tools of medicine into this paradigm means allocating these tools to those places where they will do the most good and the least harm. It also means aligning this process with the larger goals of our society.

For example, if we truly wish, as is often intoned in commercials and fund-raising events, to "end cancer in our lifetime," we will not allow for the majority of our cancer research funds to go into detection and treatment programs to the exclusion of efforts to address and correct the well-known preventable causes of cancer. This will require a collaboration of medical and non-medical fields. This collaboration is not happening today because we operate on an exclusively Anti-Trust model. Trust, then, is also about assigning tasks to those whose gifts are best suited to the task. It is about assigning our personal resources to those avenues which yield the greatest results for us. Making that kind of decision is a little easier when you realize that you actually have the ability to fix a sprained ankle, to cleanse your body of toxins, to perform an act as simple as running, or as complex and miraculous as giving birth, without submitting yourself to an "expert" or relying on technology to ensure success.

Contextualizing medicine and De-Pathologizing the body presents an important imperative upon the individual to take proactive steps. For some, this is a challenge, not simply because it is human nature to procrastinate but also because a kind of stoic self-reliance may be a culturally learned ethic.

As a male growing up in New England, I was always acutely aware of a cultural expectation of what I perceived as a manly attitude toward my body which to me seemed to celebrate men based on their ability to ignore their body's signals, especially the uncomfortable ones. I grew up running barefoot across frozen lakes, wearing tee shirts in below zero days, and embracing the physical pain of life as a track and long distance runner. And while there is much to be said for the mental fortitude that develops in such environments, I nevertheless found myself in a deep conflict when my mentors in chiropractic school informed me that if I was to become a healer, I would have to develop my body as an instrument of and for health. That meant getting adjusted regularly, even if I was not in pain. It meant massage, meditation, healthy diet, and emotional and psychological inquiry. It meant devoting resources to myself. As a Vermont man, I interpreted my highest role as the person who should be willing to sacrifice his own needs for the needs of others. These well-being measures felt like "pampering." It took some time for me to realize that, while I needed to keep the mental fortitude and toughness that growing up a short, skinny kid in New England had fostered, I now needed to develop the toughness to foster within myself a state of health and well-being that required a whole different kind of courage.

Ultimately, I knew I needed to re-design my own mythology around being a man. This new mythology must integrate what I now knew to be true about manliness: that ignoring my inner self, physical, mental, emotional, or spiritual was actually a cop-out, and that I was no good to anyone as a healer (or as a person) as long as I continued to avoid confronting my own development as a multi-dimensional being.

This misplaced courage applies to women just as much. I have moms who come into the office who have sacrificed so much of themselves in caring for their children that they have become their child's greatest obstacle to well-being. The mom herself is undernourished, under-rested, overworked and, worst of all, bitter and resentful. A very effective teaching tool, if something of a bromide, is the oxygen mask analogy. I remind them that, on the airplane, when the flight attendant explains the air bag procedures, he or she emphasizes that "if you are traveling with a small child, be sure to place the oxygen mask on YOURSELF FIRST, then help the child." Though in an emergency one can imagine oneself rushing to help the child first, you can also imagine the danger: if you lose consciousness, there is no one to help the child.

At its core, Trust is about just that. Trust. Not a blind trust that everything will always turn out all right and nothing needs to be done. We know that everything does not always turn out all right. There are times we need to be saved, we need help, heroic intervention. If I am injured in a car accident and have massive bleeding and internal trauma, I do not want a chiropractor in that moment. I want a trained medical doctor and all the technology that is available: drugs, surgery, even the machine that goes "beep!" And in that moment, I want a doctor like my father in law, who in medical emergencies trusts *nothing*. Trust, in those moments, can be a deadly liability. Emergency, life-saving intervention, end stage organ disease, and other immediate, urgent threats to life are where allopathic medicine shines, and we are so incredibly fortunate to have the incredible advances and technologies available to us in this field, in those moments.

But, unless I am a very, very reckless driver, I am not in a major car accident every day. Those cases are the exception, not the rule. The rest of the time involves moments, situations, experiences where applying that same "Anti-Trust" mentality is a liability, not an asset. For most of our lives, our bodies are the very model of "Trustworthiness," and aligning ourselves with that potential drives the choices that we make and the destiny we bring to ourselves, our world, and all the future generations to come.

Inroads have been made towards debunking the *Born Broken* philosophy.

Breast Cancer awareness month in October has always been a frustrating time for me, since I know that the majority of the resources and information gleaned from these efforts are directed towards costly and damaging diagnosis and treatment initiatives rather than anything close to prevention. However, recently I followed a link prompt called "Reduce Risks for Breast Cancer" and discovered a little video by Dr. Marissa Weiss, founder of BreastCancer.org, who spends the next three and a half minutes talking about lifestyle practices that can help reduce your actual risk of developing breast cancer, like:

- Maintaining a healthy weight
- Exercising 5-7 hours per week
- Reducing alcohol, smoking, and red meat
- Consuming organic fruits and vegetables, especially from the "Dirty Dozen" category
- Using natural housecleaning products
- Fragrance-free beauty products

This information still represents the minority of public health measures promoted in the U.S. relating to cancer, but it is a step in the right direction.

Wellbeing initiatives like the one at the University of Minnesota mentioned briefly in Chapter 1 are great examples of proactive measures that address the roots of health and wellness that truly define the "rule" of our human lives, rather than just the "exception." At their Center for Spirituality & Healing, individuals are empowered to learn, engage, and take action towards enhancing their Wellbeing, based on a model of Wellbeing that is not only multi-dimensional—

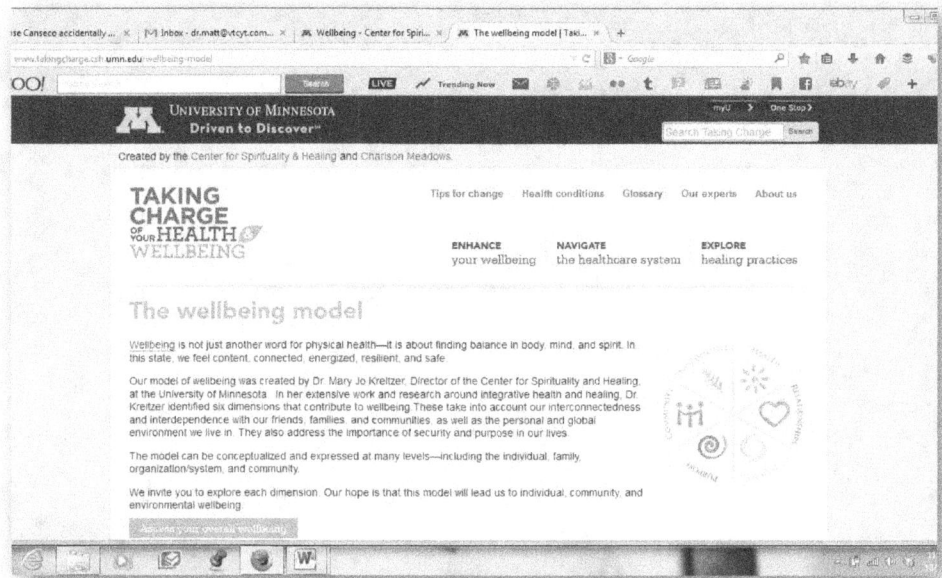

integrating the concepts of balance between mental, emotional, and physical health—but also takes into consideration the importance of our relationships to ourselves, to others, and even to our environment. The importance of security, financial and psychological, as well as purpose, is stressed in this model.

Participants are encouraged to explore and take action with a complex network of access points for a wide variety of healing practices:

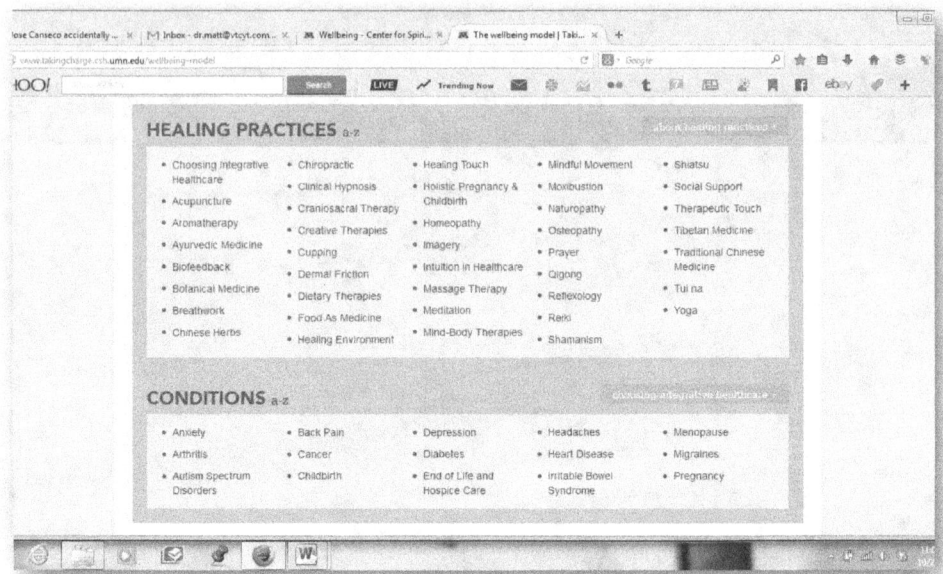

With all we know about the complex, multidimensional nature of wellness, this model is a huge step forward in the reconciliation of the two realms of health and health care. The stark contrast to our current system of incentivizing the most expensive and last-minute interventions is glaring.

One of the biggest obstacles that I have seen in my patients taking full control of their health and making positive choices toward their well-being is the subtle influence of Pathologization in their paradigm of health. Pathologization internalizes the source of illness and externalizes the source of health. Thus the goal of this book has been to deconstruct the paradigm of Pathologization in order to liberate a space within the mind of the reader that accommodates another paradigm: Trust. In the Trust paradigm, the source of health is within and the source of illness is without, in the sense that our behaviors, choices, and life experiences are the primary factors which influence our health. Health comes from within and we can either make choices and take actions that suppress or facilitate the expression of the beautiful symphony that lies within each of us.

Life in Trust is not a passive process of simply leaning back and "trusting" that our body will take care of everything. In fact, quite the opposite: The more awareness one acquires about the amazing wisdom of our bodies, the more clear it becomes that our health is like a seed deep in the soil. We must actively nurture it, water it, weed it, feed it, even as the seed remains hidden. As it sprouts and grows, its needs may change, so we must be aware, listening, watchful, and flexible, and adaptive. Intrinsic to all these faculties is a trust that if we treat this growing thing right, there is no reason why it should not express its full potential.

I have shared some personal stories of life in Trust: my first day running barefoot felt like a leap of faith. But that brings up an important distinction—it was not, in fact, a leap of faith. A leap of faith is defined as "the act of believing or accepting something intangible, unprovable, or without empirical evidence." But I had all the evidence in the world that the human body, my human body, could sustain running my feet on the ground in which my ancestors evolved (running). I had grown up spending summers outside, playing, running barefoot without thinking of it. In fact, the belief that going for a run without running shoes was an act of faith, was, itself the *real* leap of faith. I had *faith* in running shoes, not empirical evidence.

What I was engaged in was a Leap of Trust. A Leap of Trust in an act of confronting fear, not uncertainty. A Leap of Trust does not compel us to have faith in the unknown, but rather in the known. I recently did a talk on this subject and for the talk I did an internet search for "Leap of Faith" and I included these two images, which were representative of what Google provided:

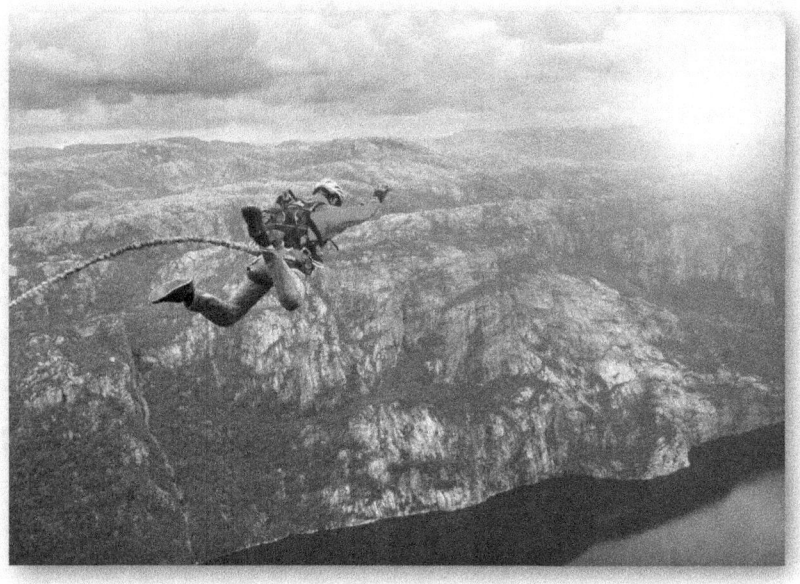

Regarding the image of the bungee jumper, we can ask the question, is this truly a leap of faith? This person has objective, tangible, provable, empirical evidence literally up the wazoo.

He has to TRUST the ropes and harness, but he does not have to have faith in them.

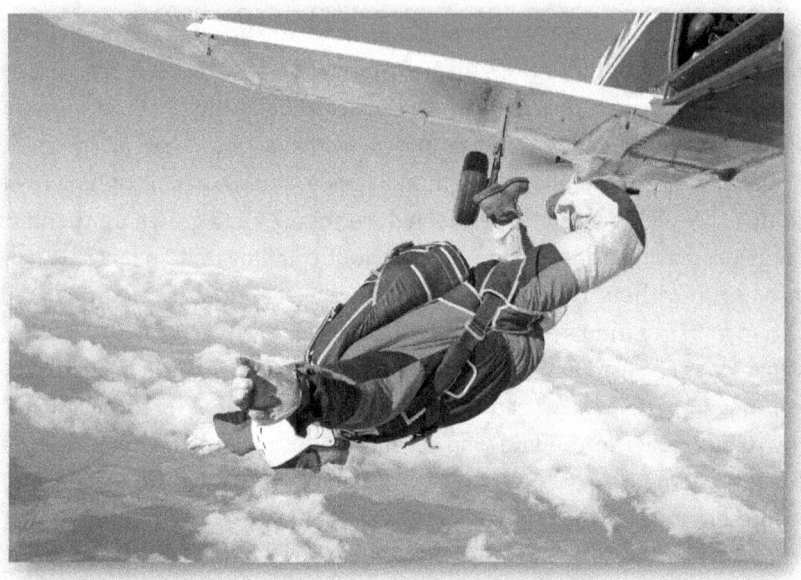

And would you jump out of a plane "in the absence of any empirical, tangible evidence" that your parachute would keep you from going splat? These are not leaps of faith. These are leaps of Trust.

Living in Trust may feel like a step into the space over a deep chasm, but in reality it is simply a willingness to recognize what is real and proven in our lives on a daily basis. In fact, many of the fears which inform the Anti-Trust paradigm are actually Leaps of Faith: believing in something without empirical evidence. It is a Leap of Faith to believe that the process responsible for the existence of every living human is intrinsically pathological. It is a Leap of Faith to believe that our bodies are incapable of healing a sprained ankle effectively without ice or Advil. Living in that kind of faith perpetually polarizes ourselves from our bodies, whereas taking Leaps of Trust engenders a relationship with ourselves which is perpetually deepening, informing, and enriching.

As a paradigm for Health and for Life, Trust is a powerful metaphor. Ultimately, Living in Trust is about connection within ourselves and with our body's intelligence.

We can trust our relationships to others, to our natural world, and to spirit. Connection is at the heart of our deepest desires, and disconnection is the fuel that energizes Pathologization. They exist in a complementary pairing, and, as in all things, the key is balance, identifying those moments when Anti-Trust is the appropriate paradigm and those in which Trust will bring better results and safely deepen our sense of connection. The first step is establishing a distinction. The next step is up to you.

ENDNOTES

1. Norwood WI, Lang P, Casteneda AR, Campbell DN. Experience with operations for hypoplastic left heart syndrome. *J Thorac Cardiovasc Surg.* Oct 1981;82(4):511-9.

2. Surgical Treatment of Pediatric Hypoplastic Left Heart Syndrome. Medscape website. http://emedicine.medscape.com/article/904137-overview. Published 1999. Updated April 11, 2014. Last accessed April 25, 2016.

3. U.S Health Care Hits $3 Trillion. Forbes website. www.forbes.com/sites/danmunro/2012/01/19/u-s-healthcare-hits-3-trillion/ Published January 19, 2012. Last accessed April 25, 2016.

4. Becker's ASC review leigh page. http://www.beckersasc.com/news-analysis/healthcare-spending-reaches-173-of-gnp-largest-1-year-rise-ever-recorded.html. Published Feb. 4, 2010. Last accessed April 25, 2016.

5. Oxford Dictionary website http://oxforddictionaries.com/definition/english/medicine?q=medicine. Last modified April 25, 2016. Last accessed April 25, 2016.

6. Medical School Curriculum Chart. Emory University website http://med.emory.edu/documents/4%20Year%20Curriculum%20Table.pdf Last modified March 26, 2013. Last accessed April 26, 2016.

7. UT Southwestern Medical Center website http://www.utsouthwestern.edu/education/medical-school/academics/curriculum/electives.html. Modified April 26, 2016. Last accessed April 25, 2016.

8. Vickie Iovine, *The Girlfriend's Guide to Pregnancy* (New York: Pocket Books,1995):71.

9. Mitang, H. Death of a President: A 200 Year Old Malpractice Debate. *New York Times.* December 14, 1999. http://www.nytimes.com/1999/12/14/health/death-of-a-president-a-200-year-old-malpractice-debate.html. Last accessed April 25, 2016.

10. Starr, P *The Social Transformation of American Medicine.* (New York: Basic Books, 1982):82

11. Starr, *The Social Transformation of American Medicine*, 95

12. Starr, *The Social Transformation of American Medicine*, 112

13. Starr, *The Social Transformation of American Medicine*, 91

14. Starr, *The Social Transformation of American Medicine*, 111

15. Starr, *The Social Transformation of American Medicine*, 100

16. Starr, *The Social Transformation of American Medicine*, 140

17. Helmuth, L. Why Are You Not Dead Yet? Slate website. http://www.slate.com/articles/health_and_science/science_of_longevity/2013/09/life_expectancy_history_public_health_and_medical_advances_that_lead_to.html   Published September 25, 2013. Updated April 25, 2016. Last accessed April 25, 2016.

18. Helmuth, L. Why Are You Not Dead Yet? Slate website. http://www.slate.com/articles/health_and_science/science_of_longevity/2013/09/life_expectancy_history_public_health_and_medical_advances_that_lead_to.html   Published September 25, 2013. Updated April 25, 2016. Last accessed April 25, 2016.

19. McKeown, T *The Origins of Human Disease.* (Cambridge MA: Basil Blackwell, 1988): 81.

20. McKinley, JB and McKinley, SM. The questionable contribution of medical measures to the decline of mortality in the United States in the twentieth century. *Health and Society.* The Milibank Memorial Fund Quarterly;1977;55:405-28.

21. Starr, *The Social Transformation of American Medicine*, 140

22. Lipman, F. Changing Our Disease Care System to a Health Care System. Huffington Post. August 15, 2010. http://www.huffingtonpost.com/dr-frank-lipman/changing-our-disease-care_b_453743.html. Last accessed April 25, 2016

23. *Taber's Cyclopedic Medical Dictionary. 16th Ed.* (Philadelphia: F.A. Davis Co,1985): 784

24. Riekman, G. *Make Your Life Extraordinary: The Power of One* [audio file]. www.LIFE.edu.

25. Chronic Illness and Mental Health. National Institute of Mental Health website. http://www.nimh.nih.gov/health/publications/depression-and-heart-disease/index.shtml. Modified April 25, 2016. Last accessed April 25, 2016.

26. Ornish, D *Dr. Dean Ornish's Program for Reversing Heart Disease.* (New York: Ballantine Books, 1990) :89.

27. Ornish, D *Dr. Dean Ornish's Program for Reversing Heart Disease*, 91.

28. Health-Related Quality of Life. Centers for Disease3 Control and Prevention website. http://www.cdc.gov/hrqol/wellbeing.htm#three. Updated April 25, 2016. Last accessed April 25, 2016.

29. Well-Being. University of Minnesota website. http://www.csh.umn.edu/wellbeing/index.html. Published July 15, 2015. Updated April 25, 2016. Last accessed April 25, 2016.

30. Taylor, S. Out of the Darkness: The Science of Post-Traumatic Growth. Psychology Today website. https://www.psychologytoday.com/blog/out-the-darkness. Updated April 25, 2016. Last accessed April 25, 2016.

31. Profiles in Health: Edward Bergmark. MPR news website. March 31, 2014. http://www.mprnews.org/story/2014/03/31/healthy-states-edward-bergmark. Last accessed April25, 2016.

32. Weil, A. U.S. Manages Disease, Not Health. CNN news website. Published March 10, 2013. http://www.cnn.com/2013/03/08/opinion/weil-health-care. Last accessed April 25, 2016.

33. Oxford Dictionary website. http://oxforddictionaries.com/definition/english/medicine?q=medicine. Last accessed April 25, 2016.

34. Zipes, DP, Wellens, HJ. Sudden Cardiac Death. *Circulation.* 1998;98;2334-2351

35. Asymptomatic Cancer. Cancer-Symptoms.com website. September 3, 2012. http://www.cancer-symptoms.com/asymptomatic-cancer-2/. Updated September 4, 2015. Last accessed April 25, 2016.

36. Gross, J. James F. Fixx Dies Jogging; Author on Running was 52. *New York Times.* July 22, 1984. http://www.nytimes.com/1984/07/22/obituaries/james-f-fixx-dies-jogging-author-on-running-was-52.html. Last accessed April 25, 2016.

37. Smith, S. Spur Spurns Critics. *Chicago Tribune.* March 14, 2000. http://articles.chicagotribune.com/2000-03-14/sports/0003140273_1_noel-elliott-sean-elliott-new-kidney/. Last accessed April 25, 2016.

38. Farshad F, M.D., M.P.H., Stafford R, M.D., Ph.D. *N Engl J Med.* 2012; 367:889-891. September 6, 2012. DOI: 10.1056/NEJM

39. Ornish, D *Dr. Dean Ornish's Program for Reversing Heart Disease,* 91.

40. *Taber's Cyclopedic Medical Dictionary. 16th Ed.* (Philadelphia: F.A. Davis Co,1985):440.

41. *Taber's Cyclopedic Medical Dictionary. 16th Ed.* (Philadelphia: F.A. Davis Co,1985):785

42. *Alternative Medicine,* October, 2007.

43. *American Cancer Society,* November 2007.

44. Screening for Breast Cancer with Mammography. Cochrane Review website. Published June 4, 2013. http://summaries.cochrane.org/CD001877/screening-for-breast-cancer-with-mammography#sthash.BQgXCSUT.dpuf. Modified April 21, 2016. Last accessed April 25, 2016.

45. *Alternative Medicine,* October, 2007.

46. World Cancer Research Fund website. Worldwide Data, 2012. *http://www.wcrf.org/cancer_statistics/world_cancer_statistics.php.* Last accessed May 1, 2016.

47. *Across the Fence,* Vermont Public Television, 2001

48. *American Cancer Society*, November 2007.

49. National Ovarian Cancer Coalition website. Can Ovarian Cancer be Prevented? http://www.ovarian.org/prevention.php. Last accessed May 1, 2016.

50. "The results of population studies to examine associations between oral contraceptive use and cancer risk have not always been consistent. Overall, however, the risks of endometrial and ovarian cancer appear to be reduced with the use of oral contraceptives, whereas the risks of breast, cervical, and liver cancer appear to be increased." *American Journal of Obstetrics and Gynecology* 2004; 190(4 Suppl):S5–22, cited by National Cancer Institute at the National Institute of Health (http://www. cancer.gov/cancertopics/factsheet/Risk/oral-contraceptives) September 26, 2013.

51. President's Cancer Panel. Reducing Environmental Cancer Risk. *Annual Report.* 2008-2009. US Department of Health and Human Services, National Institutes of Health, National Cancer Institute, April 2010.

52. Doll R and Peto R. The causes of cancer: quantitative estimates of avoidable risks of cancer in the United States today. Journal of the National Cancer Institute 1981;66:1191-1308; Doll R. Epidemiological evidence of the effects of behavior and the environment on the risk of human cancer. *Recent Results in Cancer Research.* 1998;154:3-21.

53. Xia YQ, Zhang D, Yang CX, et al. An approach to the effect on tumors of acupuncture in combination with radiotherapy or chemotherapy. *J Tradit Chin Med* 1986;6 (1): 23-6.

54. Zhou RX, Huang FL, Jiang SR, et al. The effect of acupuncture on the phagocytic activity of human leukocytes. *J Tradit Chin Med* 1988;8 (2): 83-4.

55. He CJ, Gong KH, Xu QZ, et al. Effects of microwave acupuncture on the immunological function of cancer patients. *J Tradit Chin Med* 1987;7 (1): 9-11.

56. Wu B, Zhou RX, Zhou MS. Effect of acupuncture on interleukin-2 level and NK cell immunoactivity of peripheral blood of malignant tumor patients. *Zhongguo Zhong Xi Yi Jie He Za Zhi* 1994;14 (9): 537-9.

57. Wu B, Zhou RX, Zhou MS. Effect of acupuncture on immunomodulation in patients with malignant tumors. *Zhongguo Zhong Xi Yi Jie He Za Zhi* 1996;16(3):139-41.

58. Wei Z. Clinical observation on therapeutic effect of acupuncture at zusanli for leukopenia. *J Tradit Chin Med* 1998;18(2): 94-5.

59. Ye F, Chen S, Liu W. Effects of electro-acupuncture on immune function after chemotherapy in 28 cases. *J Tradit Chin Med* 2002;22(1): 21-3.

60. Teodorczyk-Injeyan, J, Injeyan, S, Ruegg, R. Spinal Manipulative Therapy Reduces Inflammatory Cytokines but Not Substance P Production in Normal Subjects. *J Manipulative Physiol Ther.* 2006 (Jan); 29(1):14–21.

61. Selano, J.; Hightower, B.; Pfleger, B.; Collins, K.; Grostic, J.The Effects of Specific Upper Cervical Adjustments on the CD4 Counts of HIV Positive Patients. *Chiropractic Research J.* 1994; 3(1): 32–39

62. Mercola, J. Do You Take Any of these 11 Dangerous Statins or Cholesterol Drugs? Mercola website. July 20, 2010. http://articles.mercola.com/sites/articles/archive/2010/07/20/the-truth-about-statin-drugs-revealed.aspx. Updated April 26, 2016. Last accessed April 26, 2016.

63. Abramson, J and Redberg, R. Don't Give Patients More Statins. *New York Times.* November 13, 2013. http://www.nytimes.com/2013/11/14/opinion/dont-give-more-patients-statins.html?_r=0. Modified April 26, 2016. Last accessed April 26, 2016.

64. Mercola, J. New Bombshell of Disastrous Side Effects of Stains... Mercola website June 12, 2010. http://articles.mercola.com/sites/articles/archive/2010/06/12/unintended-statin-sideeffect-risks-uncovered.aspx. Modified April 26, 2016. Last accessed April 26, 2016.

65. Best Care at Lower Cost: The Path to Continuously Learning Health Care in America. National Academies of Science, Engineering and Medicine web site. September 6, 2012. http://iom.edu/Reports/2012/Best-Care-at-Lower-Cost-The-Path-to-Continuously-Learning-Health-Care-in-America.aspx. Last modified August 19, 2015. Last accessed April 26, 2016.

66. Best Care at Lower Cost: The Path to Continuously Learning Health Care in America. National Academies of Science, Engineering and Medicine web site. September 6, 2012. http://iom.edu/Reports/2012/Best-Care-at-Lower-Cost-The-Path-to-Continuously-Learning-Health-Care-in-America.aspx. Last modified August 19, 2015. Last accessed April 26, 2016.

67. Nordqvist, C. U.S. Healthcare System Squanders $750 Billion a Year. <u>Medical News Today September 7, 2012</u> http://www.medicalnewstoday.com/articles/249970.php. Last accessed April 26, 2016.

68. Mangan, D. Medical Bills Are the Biggest Cause of U.S. Bankruptcies: Study. CNBC web site. Tuesday, 25 June 2013 http://www.cnbc.com/id/100731877. Last modified July 24, 2013. Last accessed April 26, 2016.

69. *Deadly Delivery: The Maternal Health Care Crisis in the USA.* Amnesty International Publications. 2010; ISBN # 978-0-86210-458-0

70. Is U.S. Health Really the Best in the World? *JAMA.* 2000;284(4):483-485. doi:10.1001/jama.284.4.483

71. Is U.S. Health Really the Best in the World? *JAMA.* 2000;284(4):483-485. doi:10.1001/jama.284.4.483

72. Flockhart D, MD, PhD, Honig P, MD, MPH, Usdin Yasuda S, MS, PharmD, Rosebraugh C, MD, MPH, Centers for Education and Research on Therapeutics Lecture Guide, *Preventable Adverse Drug Reactions:A Focus on Drug Interactions.* http://www.azcert.org/medical-pros/education/CERT%20Lecture%20Guide.pdf. Accessed October 1, 2013.

73. Tavernise, S. Ohio County Losing its Young to Painkiller's Grip. *New York Times.* April 19, 2011. http://www.nytimes.com/2011/04/20/us/20drugs.html?nl=todays headlines&emc=tha23&_r=0. Accessed April 26, 2016.

74. Mercola, D. One in Four Over 45 Take this Unnecessary Drug. Mercola website. May 9, 2009. http://articles.mercola.com/sites/articles/archive/2011/05/09/one-in-four-over-45-take-this-unnecessary-drug.aspx. Last accessed April 26, 2016.

75. Retail Prescription Drugs Filled At Pharmacies (Annual Per Capita By Age). The Henry J. Kaiser Family Foundation website. 2015. http://kff.org/other/state-indi-cator/retail-rx-drugs-by-age/. Last accessed April 26, 2016.

76. Makary, M. How to Stop Hospitals From Killing Us. *The Wall Street Journal* September 21, 2012. http://www.wsj.com/articles/SB10000872396390444620104 578008263334441352. Last accessed April 26, 2016.

77. Healthcare Consumerism and Hospital Quality in America Report. HealthGrades. 2011 http://www.heatlhgrades.com/business/img/healthcareconsumerismhos-pitalqualityreport2011.pdf Last accessed June 14, 2016.

78. *Newsweek*. Sept 24, 2012.

79. *Doctored*. Jeff Hayes Film. Working pictures, 2012.

80. *Health Aff 10.1377/hlthaff.2010.0073*; published ahead of print October 7, 2010.

81. *Health Aff 10.1377/hlthaff.2010.0073*; published ahead of print October 7, 2010.

82. Best Care at Lower Cost: The Path to Continuously Learning Health Care in America. National Academies of Science, Engineering and Medicine web site. September 6, 2012. http://iom.edu/Reports/2012/Best-Care-at-Lower-Cost-The-Path-to-Continuously-Learning-Health-Care-in-America.aspx. Last modified August 19, 2015. Last accessed April 26, 2016.

83. Boyles, S. More U.S. Deaths from MRSA than AIDS. *WebMD* website. October 16, 2007. http://www.webmd.com/skin-problems-and-treatments/news/20071016/more-us-deaths-from-mrsa-than-aids. Last accessed April 27, 2016.

84. Andrews, RM. *The National Hospital Bill: The Most Expensive Conditions by Payer, 2006*. Healthcare Cost and Utilization Project, Statistical Brief, 59, 2008:7; www.hcup-us.ahrq.gov/reports/statbriefs/sb59.pdf. Last accessed April 27, 2016.

85. Maternal Mortality in 2005. WHO, UNICEF, UNFPA and The World Bank. http://www.who.int/whosis/mme_2005.pdf. Last accessed April 27, 2016.

86. Rosenthal, E. American Way of Birth: Costliest in the World. *New York Times,* June 30, 2013. http://www.nytimes.com/2013/07/01/health/american-way-of-birth-costliest-in-the-world.html?pagewanted=all&_r=0. Last accessed April 27, 2016.

87. *Business of Being Born,* Abby Epstein, Ricki Lake. New Line Cinemas, 2008.

88. Edwards, K. *Memory Keeper's Daughter.* New York: Penguin Books, 2005:9.

89. Goldsmith, J. Traditional Childbirth. *Mothering Magazine,* Spring, 1989.

90. Arms, S. *Immaculate Deception II.* Berkeley CA: Celestial Arts Press,1994:42

91. Health in America. City University of New York website. http://www.cuny.edu/archive/cc/health-in-america/public-health.html. Last accessed May 14, 2015.

92. Health in America. City University of New York website. http://www.cuny.edu/archive/cc/health-in-america/public-health.html. Last accessed May 14, 2015.

93. Health in America. City University of New York website. http://www.cuny.edu/archive/cc/health-in-america/public-health.html. Last accessed May 14, 2015.

94. Centers for Disease Control and Prevention website. www.CDC.gov

95. Shorter, E. *A History of Women's Bodies.* New York: Penguin Books, 1982:3

96. Shorter, E. *A History of Women's Bodies,* 2

97. Shorter, E. *A History of Women's Bodies,*7

98. Shorter, E. *A History of Women's Bodies,* 23

99. Weick, M. A History of Rickets in the United States. *American Journal of Clinical Nutrition,* vol. 20, No.11, Nov 1967:1234-1241.100

100. Bills, CE. Physiology of the Sterols, *Physiol.* Rev. 15: 1, 1935.

101. Shorter, E. *A History of Women's Bodies*, 28

102. Dundes, L. The Evolution of the Maternal Birthing Position.*AJPH* May 1987 Vol 77 No. 5.

103. Dundes, L. The Evolution of the Maternal Birthing Position.*AJPH* May 1987 Vol 77 No. 5.

104. Dundes, L. The Evolution of the Maternal Birthing Position.*AJPH* May 1987 Vol 77 No. 5.

105. Mauriceau F. The Diseases of Women with Child and in Child-Bed. London: John Darby, 1863 (original work published in French in 1668).

106. Dundes, L. The Evolution of the Maternal Birthing Position.*AJPH* May 1987 Vol 77 No. 5.

107. Thompson, WI, *The Time Falling Bodies Take to Light.* NY: St. Martin's Press, 1981 :9

108. Ganme JP, Carson CC. Frère Jacques Beaulieu: from rogue lithotomist to nursery rhyme character. *J Urol. April 1999*;161(4):1067-9.

109. Dundes, L. The Evolution of the Maternal Birthing Position.*AJPH* May 1987 Vol 77 No. 5.

110. Davis-Floyd, R. The Rituals of American Hospital Birth. April 11, 2014. *http://davis-floyd.com/uncategorized/the-rituals-of-american-hospital-birth-2/*. Last accessed April 27, 2016.

111. Caldeyro-Barcia, R. qtd in O'Mara, P, Facciolo, J, and Ponet, W. 2003. *Mothering Magazine's Having a Baby, Naturally: The Mothering Magazine Guide to Pregnancy and Childbirth.* Simon and Shuster.

112. Dundes, L. The Evolution of the Maternal Birthing Position.*AJPH* May 1987 Vol 77 No. 5.

113. Leavitt, J. Joseph B. DeLee and the Practice of Preventive Obstetrics. *Am J Public Health,* 1988 October; 78(10): 1353–1361.

114. Bynum, W. *History of Medicine.* NY: Oxford University Press, 2008:43

115. Arms, S. *Immaculate Deception II*, Berkeley CA: Celestial Arts Press,1994: 56.

116. Hooker, R, M.D. *Maternal Mortality in New York City - A Study of all Puerperal Deaths, 1930-1932.* NY: The Commonwealth Fund: 1933.

117. Loudon, I. *Death in Childbirth: An International Study of Maternal Care and Maternal Mortality 1800-1950.* Oxford: Clarendon Press: 1993.

118. Loudon, I. *Death in Childbirth: An International Study of Maternal Care and Maternal Mortality 1800-1950.* Oxford: Clarendon Press: 1993.

119. Shorter E. *A History of Women's Bodies,* 127

120. Historical and statistical data from this section derived primarily from Nuland, S. Doctors: The Biography of Medicine. New York: Vintage Books, 1988: Chapter 9, *The Germ Theory Before Germs: The Enigma of Ignaz Semmelweis.*

121. Nuland, S. *Doctors,* 240

122. Nuland, S. *Doctors,* 240

123. Nuland, S. *Doctors,* 240

124. Nuland, S. *Doctors,* 248

125. Holmes, O. (1809–1894) reprinted *Arch Dis Child Fetal Neonatal Ed.* Jul 2007; 92(4): F325–F327.

126. Meigs C D. Females and their diseases: a series of letters to his Class. Philadelphia: Lea and Blanchard:1848.

127. Hodge H L. On the non-contagious character of puerperal fever: an introductory lecture. Philadelphia: TK & PG Collins, 1852.

128. Hodge H L. On the non-contagious character of puerperal fever: an introductory lecture. Philadelphia: TK & PG Collins, 1852.

129. Nuland, S. *Doctors,* 245

130. Nuland, S. *Doctors,* 245

131. Loudon, I Maternal Mortality in the Past and its Relevance to Developing Countries Today. *Am J Clin Nutr* July 2000 *vol. 72 no. 1 241s-246s*

132. RCM Midwives. November 2002;5(11):370-1.

133. Wagner, M. *Born in the USA,* Los Angeles, CA: University of California Press, 2006:9.

134. Gaskin, IM, *Birth Matters.* NY: Seven Stories Press; 2011:74.

135. Wertz, R and D. *Lying-In: A History of Childbirth in America.* NY: The Free Press,1977:9.

136. Gaskin, IM, *Birth Matters,* 73

137. DeClerq, E The Trials of Hannah Porn: The Campaign to Abolish Midwifery in Massachussetts. *American Journal of Public Health* June 1984 Vol. 84 No. 6 [http://www.ncbi.nlm.nih.gov/pmc/articles/PMC1614962/pdf/amjph00457-0144.pdf] Accessed May 1, 2016.

138. Gaskin, IM, *Birth Matters,* 81

139. Gaskin, IM, *Birth Matters,* 80

140. Gaskin, IM, *Birth Matters,* 78

141. Kahn, R. *Bearing Meaning: The Language of Birth,* Chicago: University of Illinois Press, 1995:191.

142. Kahn, R. *Bearing Meaning: The Language of Birth,*:192

143. Gibson, F The Official Plan to Eliminate the Midwife: 1900-1930. Modified September 8, 2012 [http://www.collegeofmidwives.org/collegeofmidwives.org/safety_issues01/rosenbl1.htm. Last accessed May 1, 2016.

144. Loudon, I Maternal Mortality in the Past and its Relevance to Developing Countries Today. *Am J Clin Nutr* July 2000 *vol. 72 no. 1 241s-246s*

145. *Surgery, Gynecology, and Obstetrics*, Volume 34 (January to June 1922).

146. http://www.collegeofmidwives.org/collegeofmidwives.org/safety_issues01/rosenbl1.htm

147. http://www.collegeofmidwives.org/collegeofmidwives.org/safety_issues01/rosenbl1.htm

148. Ehrenreich, B and English, D. *Witches, Midwives and Nurses: A History of Women Healers.* (New York: The Feminist Press; 1973).

149. Arms, S. *Immaculate Deception II*, Berkeley CA: Celestial Arts Press,1994:44

150. Ehrenreich, B and English, D. *Witches, Midwives and Nurses: A History of Women Healers.* New York: The Feminist Press; 1973.

151. Blumenfeld-Kozinski. *Not of Woman Born: Representations of Caesarian Birth in Medieval and Rennaisance Culture,* Ithaca: Cornell University Press, 1990.

152. *CDC MMWR* Weekly October 01, 1999 / 48(38);849-858

153. Kahn, R. *Bearing Meaning: The Language of Birth*, Chicago: University of Illinois Press,1995:190, quoting historian Nancy Schrom Dye.

154. Achievements in Public Health, *CDC MMWR* Weekly October 01, 1999 / 48(38);849-858

155. Shorter, E. *A History of Women's Bodies*, 156

156. DeLee, J. The prophylactic forceps operation, *Am J Obstet Gynecol*. 1920;1:34-44.

157. *Am J Public Health*. October 1988; 78(10): 1353–1361. *Am J Clin Nutr.* July 2000 *vol. 72 no. 1 241s-246s.*

158. Hooker, RS, M.D. *Maternal Mortality in New York City, A Study of All Puerperal Deaths 1930-1932.* (New York, Commonwealth Fund Oxford University Press: 1933).

159. Dundes, L. The Evolution of the Maternal Birthing Position.*AJPH* May 1987 Vol 77 No. 5.

160. Sinha P, Langford K. Forceps delivery in 21st century obstetrics. *The Internet Journal of Gynecology and Obstetrics.* 2009 Volume 11 Number 2. DOI: 10.5580/239e –.

161. National Institutes of Health, U.S. National Library of Medicine. Assisted Delivery With Forceps. http://www.nlm.nih.gov/medlineplus/ency/patientin-structions/000509.htm. Modified April 15, 2016. Last accessed April 29, 2016.

162. Menticoqlou, SM, Perlman, M, Manning, FA. High Cervical Spinal Cord Injury in Neonates Delivered With Forceps. *Obstet Gynecol.* 1995 Oct;86(4 Pt 1):589-94.

163. DeLee, J. The Prophylactic Forceps Operation. *Am J Obstet Gynecol* 1920;1:34-44.

164. Hartmann, K, Viswanathan, M, Palmieri, et. al. Outcomes of Routine Episiotomy: A Systematic Review. *JAMA.* 2005 May 4;293(17):2141-8.

165. Shorter, E. *A History of Women's Bodies*, 148

166. Shorter, E. *A History of Women's Bodies*, 148

167. Wertz, R and D. *Lying-In: A History of Childbirth in America,* 150

168. Wertz, R and D. *Lying-In: A History of Childbirth in America,* 150

169. Arms, S. *Immaculate Deception II*, 78

170. Arms, S. *Immaculate Deception II*, 78

171. Dunn, H. Vital Statistics of the United States, 1955. Modified September 20, 2005. http://www.nber.org/vital-stats-books/VSUS_1955_1.CV.pdf. Last accessed April 29, 2016.

172. DeLee, J. The Prophylactic Forceps Operation. *Am J Obstet Gynecol* 1920;1:34-44.

173. *Am J Public Health*. October 1988; 78(10): 1353–1361; *Am J Clin Nutr.* July 2000 *vol. 72 no. 1 241s-246s*

174. Margulis, J. *The Business of Baby* NY: Scribner Press; 2013: 49

175. Wertz, R and D. *Lying-In: A History of Childbirth in America*, 161

176. Wertz, R and D. *Lying-In: A History of Childbirth in America*, 3

177. Achievements in Public Health, 1900-1999: Healthier Mothers and Babies. Centers for Disease Control and Prevention website. October 1, 1999. Last modified April 29, 2016. *http://www.cdc.gov/mmwr/preview/mmwrhtml/mm4838a2. htm.* Last accessed April 29, 2016.

178. Wagner, M. *Born in the USA*, 68

179. Osterman, M. and Martin, J. Epidural and Spinal Anesthesia Use During Labor: 27-State Reporting Area, 2008. National Vital Statistics Report, April 6, 2011 Vol.59 No.5 http://www.cdc.gov/nchs/data/nvsr/nvsr59/nvsr59_05.pdf. Accessed April 29, 2016.

180. Sakala, C and Correy M. *Evidence-Based Maternity: What it is and What it can Achieve.* Milibank Memorial Fund: 2008.

181. Block, J. *Pushed.* Cambridge, MA: DeCapo Press, 2007:33.

182. Sakala, C. and Correy, M. *Evidence-Based Maternity: What it is and What it can Achieve.* Milibank Memorial Fund: 2008.

183. Block, J. *Pushed,* 56

184. *Lancet* 1985; 2: 436-7.

185. Fast Stats, Centers for Disease Control and Prevention website. cdc.gov; http://www.cdc.gov/nchs/fastats/delivery.htm. Last accessed May 1, 2016.

186. Sakala, C. and Correy, M. *Evidence-Based Maternity:* (referencing Renz-Polster et al. 2005; Salam et al. 2006).

187. Sakala, C. and Correy, M. *Evidence-Based Maternity:* (referencing Penders, et al. 2006).

188. Sakala, C. and Correy, M. *Evidence-Based Maternity:* (referencing Jain and Eaton 2006).

189. Block, J. *Pushed,* 49

190. Sakala, C. and Correy, M. *Evidence-Based Maternity*

191. Margulis, J. *The Business of Baby,* 81

192. Sakala, C. and Correy, M. *Evidence-Based Maternity*

193. Margulis, J. *The Business of Baby,* 89

194. Beyond too little, too late and too much, too soon: a pathway towards evidence-based, respectful maternity care worldwide Miller, Suellen et al.The Lancet , Volume 0 , Issue 0

195. Sakala, C. and Correy, M. *Evidence-Based Maternity*

196. 196Rosenthal, E. American Way of Birth: Costliest in the World. *New York Times*, June 30, 2013. http://www.nytimes.com/2013/07/01/health/american-way-of-birth-costliest-in-the-world.html?pagewanted=all&_r=0. Last accessed April 27, 2016.

197. Cheyney, M., Bovbjerg, M., Everson, C., Gordon, W., Hannibal, D. and Vedam, S. (2014), Outcomes of Care for 16,924 Planned Home Births in the United States: The Midwives Alliance of North America Statistics Project, 2004 to 2009. Journal of Midwifery & Women's Health, 59: 17–27. doi: 10.1111/jmwh.12172

198. Margulis, J. *The Business of Baby*, 92

199. Ohm, J., Is the Pit Bull? Makin' Miracles web site, 2009. http://www.makinmiracles.com/articles_pregnancy/is_the_pit_bull.html. Modified November 10, 2015. Last accessed April 29, 2016.

200. http://www.childbirthconnection.org/article.asp?ck=10450

201. Sakala, C. and Correy, M. *Evidence-Based Maternity*

202. Wagner, M. *Born in the USA*, 75

203. McKay, S, R.N., PhD. Maternal Position During Labor and Birth: A Reassessment. *Journal of Obstetric, Gynecologic, & Neonatal Nursing.* September 1980: 288–291.

204. *Midwifery Today* E-News (Vol 1 Issue 50, Dec 10, 1999)

205. Sakala, C. and Correy, M. *Evidence-Based Maternity*

206. Sakala, C. and Correy, M. *Evidence-Based Maternity*

207. *Listening to Mothers II*

208. *Listening to Mothers II*

209. Interview, *Amherst* magazine, Spring 2010

210. Wagner, M. *Born in the USA*, 51

211. Martini, F. *Fundamentals of Anatomy and Physiology, Ninth edition*, San Francisco, CA: Pearson, 2012.

212. Wagner, M. World Health Organization "Having a Baby in Europe", European Regional Office, 1985

213. Perkins, B. *Medical Delivery Business* New Brunswick, New Jersey, Rutgers University Press: 112.

214. Moran, M. *Happy Birth Days.* Charleston, SC: Terra Publishing; 1986:24

215. With permission, Michael Scimeca, 2014.

216. *Orgasmic Birth*, copyright 2008, Sunken Treasure, LLC, directed by Debra Pascali-Bonaro.

217. House, P, Amnesty International Secretariat. *Deadly Delivery: The Maternal Care Crisis in the U.S.A.* Modified April 25, 2011 http://www.amnestyusa.org/sites/default/files/pdfs/deadlydelivery.pdf. Last accessed May 1, 2016.

218. Berg C, Danel I, Atrash H, Zane S, Bartlett L (Editors). Strategies to reduce pregnancy-related deaths: from identification and review to action. Atlanta: Centers for Disease Control and Prevention; 2001.

219. Kitzinger S and Davis J, eds. *The Place of Birth.* Oxford: Oxford University Press;1978: 62-63.

220. *Research Issues in the Assessment of Birth Settings*, Institute of Medicine, National Academy Press, Washington; 1982:76.

221. Duran AM. The safety of home birth: the farm study. *American Journal of Public Health.* 1992;82(3):450-453.

222. Home versus hospital deliveries: follow up study of matched pairs for procedures and outcome. *BMJ 1996;313:1313*

223. Otis, CH. Midwives Still Hassled by Medical Establishment. *Utne Reader*, Nov./Dec. 1990:32-34

224. Johnson Kenneth C, Daviss Betty-Anne. Outcomes of planned home births with certified professional midwives: large prospective study in North America BMJ 2005; 330 :1416

225. New York Times editorial board. Are Midwives Safer than Doctors? New York Times. December 14, 2014. http://www.nytimes.com/2014/12/15/opinion/are-midwives-safer-than-doctors.html?smid=fb-share&_r=0. Accessed May 1, 2016.

226. Janssen PA, Saxell L, Page LA, Klein MC, Liston RM, Lee Sk. Outcomes of planned home births with registered midwife versus versus planned hospital birth with midwife or physician. *CMAJ; 2009.*

227. de Jonge A, van der Goes B, Ravelli A, Amelink-Verburg M, Mol B, Nijhuis J, et al. Perinatal mortality and morbidity in a nationwide cohort of 529,688 low-risk planned home and hospital births. *BJOG; 2009.*

228. Olsen, O. Meta-Analysis of the Safety of Home Birth. *Birth 1997 Mar;24(1):4-13; discussion 14-6 Olsen O*

229. Hutton, EK, Reitsma, AH and Kaufman, K. Outcomes associated with planned home and planned hospital births in low-risk women attended by midwives in Ontario, Canada, 2003–2006: A retrospective cohort study. *Birth*, 36: 180–189. doi: 10.1111/j.1523-536X.2009.00322.x

230. Cheyney, M., Bovbjerg, M., Everson, C., Gordon, W., Hannibal, D. and Vedam, S. (2014), Outcomes of Care for 16,924 Planned Home Births in the United States: The Midwives Alliance of North America Statistics Project, 2004 to 2009. Journal of Midwifery & Women's Health, 59: 17–27. doi: 10.1111/jmwh.12172

231. Sandall J, Soltani H, Gates S, Shennan A, Devane D. Midwife-led continuity models versus other models of care for childbearing women. Cochrane Database of Systematic Reviews 2015, Issue 9. Art. No.: CD004667. DOI: 10.1002/14651858.CD004667.pub4

232. MacDorman, N., Matthews, m., and DeClerque, E., Trends in Out-of-Hospital Births in the United States, 1990-2012. Centers for Disease Control and Prevention NCHS Data Brief No. 144, March, 2014

233. Sullivan, J., Farrar, H., Fever and Antipyretic Use in Children. *Pediatrics* Vol. 127 No. 3 March 2011.

234. Thanks to the late great Dr. Ian Grassam for the LoMein/ptomaine story.

235. Bhattacharyya N, Lin HW (2010 Nov). Changes and consistencies in the epidemiology of pediatric adenotonsillar surgery. *Otolaryngol Head Neck Surg* 43(5): 680-4.

236. Mahar, M. A Blueprint for Healthcare Reform. Healthbeat Blog February 4, 2008. http://www.healthbeatblog.com/2008/02/a-blueprint-for/. Last accessed May 1, 2016.

237. Acland video dissection series, tape 6.

238. Martini, F. *Fundamentals of Anatomy and Physiology, Ninth edition*, San Francisco, CA: Pearson, 2012: 773.

239. Barras, C. Appendix Evolved More tan 30 Times. Science magazine. February 12, 2013. http://news.sciencemag.org/plants-animals/2013/02/appendix-evolved-more-30-times. Last accessed May 1, 2016.

240. Barras,C.AppendixEvolvedMoretan30Times.Sciencemagazine.February12,2013. http://news.sciencemag.org/plants-animals/2013/02/appendix-evolved-more-30-times. Last accessed May 1, 2016.

241. *SEXUALLY TRANSMITTED INFECTIONS* (London), Volume 74, Number 5; October 1998:364-367.

242. *Progrès en Urologie*, Vol. 9, No. 6, 1999:1148-1157.

243. SEXUALLY TRANSMITTED INFECTIONS (London), Volume 74, Number 5; October 1998:364-367.

244. Owings, M, Uddin, S, Williams, S. Trends in Circumcision for Male Newborns in U.S. Hospitals 1979-2010. Centers for Disease Control and Prevention. National Center for Health Statistics. Updated August 22, 2013. http://www.cdc.gov/nchs/data/ hestat/circumcision_2013/circumcision_2013.htm. Last accessed May 1, 2016.

245. Female Genital Mutilation Fact Sheet, World Health Organization Media Centre, Updated February, 2016. http://www.who.int/mediacentre/factsheets/fs241/ en/. Last accessed October 3, 2016.

246. Quotes and comments in this section refer to: McDougall, C. *Born to Run*. NY: Alfred A. Knopf, 2009.

247. Elwood, JM, Jopson, J, Melanoma and Sun Exposure: An Overview of Published Studies. *Int J Cancer*. 1997 Oct 9;73(2):198-203.

248. Evidence-based medicine: A new approach to teaching the practice of medicine. *JAMA. 1992* Nov 4;268(17):2420-5.

249. Dossey, L The Mythology of Science-Based Medicine. March 18, 2010. Updated November 17, 2011. http://www.huffingtonpost.com/dr-larry-dossey/the-mythology-of-science_b_412475.html. Last accessed May 1, 2016.

250. Jeannette Ezzo, Barker Bausell, Daniel E. Moerman, Brian Berman and Victoria Hadhazy (2001). REVIEWING THE REVIEWS. International Journal of Technology Assessment in Health Care, 17, pp 457-466.

251. Begley, S Why Almost Everything You Hear About Medicine is Wrong. *Newsweek*. Jan 24th, 2011. Last accessed May 1, 2016.

252. Engel G. The need for a new medical model: a challenge for biomedicine. *Science*. 1977;196:129–136.

253. Smith, GC, Pell, JP. Parachute use to prevent death and major trauma related to gravitational challenge: systematic review of randomised controlled trials. *BMJ.* 2003 Dec 0;327(7429):1459-61.

254. Avorn, M. Dangerous Deception- Hiding the Evidence of Adverse Drug Effects. *N Engl J Med* 2006; 355:2169-2171November 23, 2006DOI: 10.1056/*NEJM*p068246.

ABOUT THE AUTHOR

Dr. Matt Rushford is a family chiropractor, writer and educator. He has over 20 years of field experience in the areas of natural health care and natural health advocacy. He is founder and co-director of the Rushford Family Chiropractic Centers, which have served the northwestern Vermont communities since 1994. He has taught anatomy & physiology for nursing students at the Community College of Vermont since 2001 and is a member of the adjunct faculty at Johnson State College. His writing has been published in *Mothering* magazine, *Pathways for Family Wellness*, and many local and regional publications. Dr. Matt lives in Williston, Vermont with his wife Julieta, and son John Storm, and their German Shepherd, Athena. *Born Broken* is his first book.

www.ingramcontent.com/pod-product-compliance
Lightning Source LLC
Chambersburg PA
CBHW070851290526
45795CB00001B/76